KU-303-724

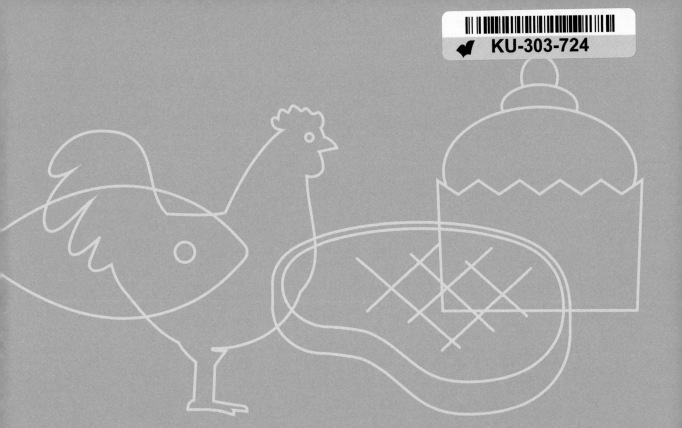

TOM KERRIDGE

LOSE WEIGHT & GET FIT

TOM KERRIDGE

LOSE WEIGHT & GET FIT

High-flavour cooking for dieting and fitness

BLOOMSBURY ABSOLUTE
LONDON • OXFORD • NEW YORK • NEW DELHI • SYDNEY

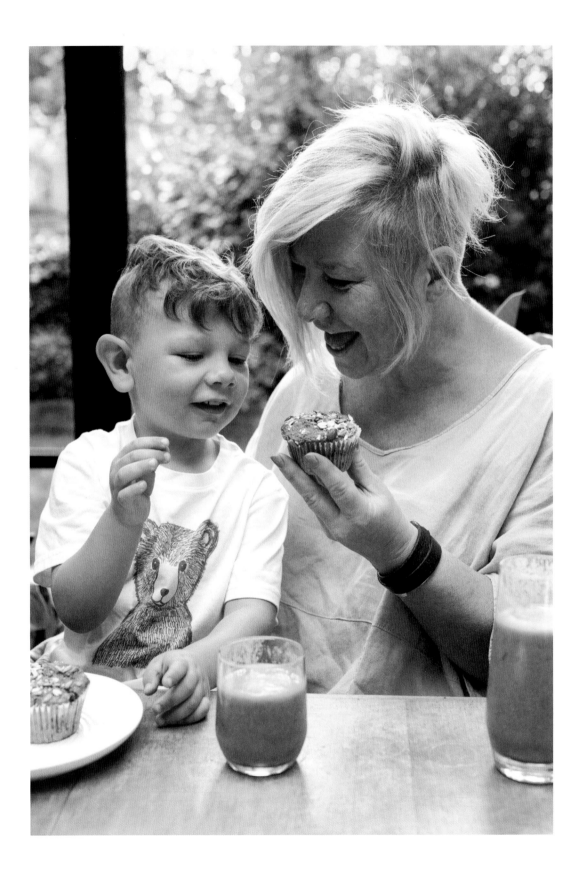

To Bef & Acey

CONTENTS

♡ Vegetarian recipes

❄ Recipes that are good for freezing

The calorie counts for recipes cannot be absolutely precise because there are many variables, including the water and fat content of ingredients, and calorie loss during cooking. The counts do, however, allow you to work out your approximate daily calorie intake.

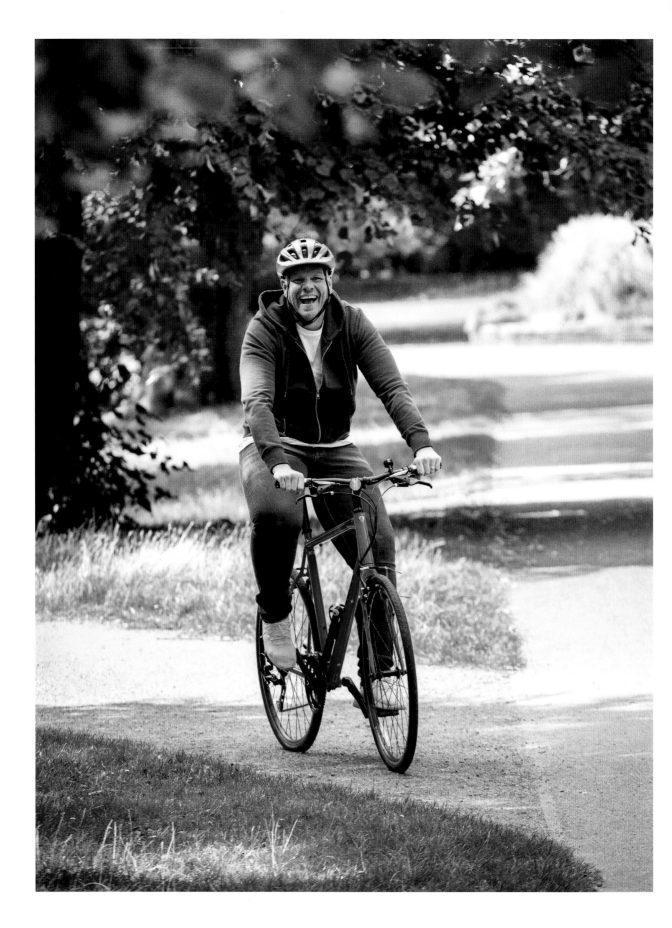

COME ON, HAVE A READ!

Five years ago, when I first set out to lose weight, I didn't really have any specific targets in mind. It was basically about wanting to be healthier and feeling fitter so I could enjoy life more. At my heaviest, I weighed around 30 stone and it wasn't easy, but I lost more than 12 stone through cutting out carbohydrates (pasta, bread, potatoes and rice) and alcohol, as well as swimming every day. I won't lie: it was bloody hard work! But it felt amazing to see such positive results.

Saying that, something important I've learned in the past couple of years is that life is not a linear journey, especially when it comes to weight loss and health. Although I'm in a lot better shape than before, I've noticed that the scales are starting to creep back up again and that my clothes aren't fitting quite the way I'd like them to any more. I could tell you the same old excuses about being busy at work, family commitments and responsibilities at home, but I know you've heard them a million times – you probably tell them to yourself! Whether I like it or not, there's no denying it: I'm heading into middle age. I may still feel like the young man who loved to party, but my body is telling me otherwise. It's now or never, and I don't want to go back to where I was.

My initial weight-loss strategy concentrated mainly on what I was eating, but now I know that it's to do with fitness as well. The food you eat directly affects your ability to stay fit, so the two working together is the secret formula for getting maximum results and maintaining those results long term. It's all about finding a way to make both of these things a priority in your life.

Fuelling fitness

You only need to look at the extreme diets of elite athletes to know that what you eat – or don't eat – can have a serious impact on performance. Now, I'm not saying we should all eat and train like Olympians, but I know from my own experience that if I've not eaten properly, working out will be that much harder. I can still hit my workout goal for the day, but it will take so much more effort to get there and I'll take longer to recover. You need to fuel yourself properly before and after exercising, and put the right things into your body.

The recipes in this book have all been calorie-counted so that you can keep an eye on your daily intake – you can work out how many calories you should be eating each day, in order to lose weight, by either using an online calculator or speaking to your doctor. They have also been put together with fitness in mind, so they contain lots of great ingredients that will help to sustain energy levels through the day and during your workout, and help your muscles recover afterwards.

Carbohydrates and protein are both vital when it comes to fuelling your body. Unrefined carbohydrates (carbohydrates in their natural, unprocessed form) will give you slow-release energy and help replace the sugars that get used up during a workout. I like ingredients such as oats, wholegrain pasta, sweet potatoes and brown rice. The 'overnight oats' on pages 24 and 26 are a great choice for refuelling after exercise: pack a portion into a food container and take it with you to eat after your morning workout. Or if you're working out in the evening, try making the chicken and yoghurt curry with rice on page 176 when you get home.

I have also included lots of lean protein in the recipes, which is really important for muscle repair after exercise. Great sources of lean protein include chicken, turkey, fish and seafood, lean mince, free-range eggs, chickpeas, beans and lentils. I also use chia seeds and quinoa, both of which are excellent sources of plant-based protein, and I love the texture that these ingredients bring to dishes. After an intense cardio session, you'll need a few more carbs, and after a strength workout, you should focus on the protein, but you ideally need some of both in every meal and the recipes in this book are built around providing this. Meals that are especially good for post-workout recovery have this symbol: POST

Of course, hydration is key! Make sure you drink enough water throughout the day and especially after exercising. Both normal dairy milk and soy milk are good choices for post-workout recovery and they have even been shown to be more effective than sports drinks. They replenish fluids, as well as providing good levels of protein, carbs and other nutrients. So why not enjoy some in one of the smoothies or shakes on pages 56–63?

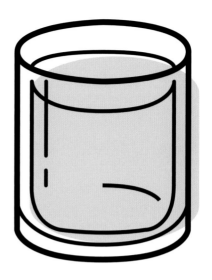

A common misconception is that because you're exercising hard you can eat more. This is true to a certain extent – especially if you don't have a lot of weight to lose. But just because you've been to the gym, it doesn't mean you can indulge in chips on the way home. Trust me, I've been there! It's true that when you're exercising you might feel a bit hungrier though, so I find it's best to time my workouts to end just before a mealtime, which means I don't end up counting down the minutes until lunch.

It also makes a difference how much time you leave between eating a meal and exercising – about 2–4 hours is a good window to aim for. My ideal time to work out is at about 11am. It means I can get a proper night's sleep, eat a good breakfast and know I will perform at my best – and then afterwards I can head straight into lunch. In reality though, I'm usually deep in work at that time, so I tend to fit exercise in either first thing in the morning or on my way home at the end of the day. If that's the case, then I'll grab something light and not too fatty, such as yoghurt and a piece of fruit, veggies dipped in hummus, toast topped with nut butter (see page 48 for my homemade recipe) or the energy balls on pages 238–243 to give me a bit of a boost beforehand.

I also try to pack in as many whole foods as I can – like fruit, veggies, whole grains and pulses such as beans and lentils – which are as close to their natural state as possible and don't contain additives. These foods are higher in fibre than processed carbs like white bread or sugary cereal, so they take longer to digest, meaning you'll feel fuller for longer. And they have the added bonus of containing loads of extra nutrients. We all know we should be avoiding cakes, sweets and crisps when we're on a diet, and that's the simple reason why: you enjoy them for the 5 minutes it takes to eat them, but then inevitably you're hungry in about an hour. So aim for more whole foods and try to stick to proper mealtimes.

If you're cutting back on meat generally, or just want to eat more veg-based meals, turn to the More Veg chapter on page 106. Also look for the ♡ symbol next to lots of the recipes, which means they're suitable for vegetarians.

Make it work for you

We all have different pulls on our time – responsibilities at home, family and work to juggle. Life is hectic and complicated. I struggle with work-life balance all the time, often working late or leaving early in the morning. That's why it is so important to find a way to make fitness and eating work properly for you and your lifestyle. There's no one-size-fits-all, so try to find some balance where you can.

According to the NHS, adults aged 19–64 should aim for 150 minutes of moderate cardio exercise (cycling, brisk walking or anything that gets your heart rate up) or 75 minutes of vigorous exercise (such as a game of tennis or running) each week. In addition, we should be doing strength exercises on two or more days a week, such as weights or activities like Pilates and yoga. That's a lot!

But if you break this down and find a way to be active every day in some way, it is much more manageable. My life doesn't really have any proper structure and so I've had to find a way to be adaptable. For me, swimming is what worked from the start. Most gyms have a pool, so it was easy for me to head down there whenever I had a spare hour, and I found I really came to enjoy it! I think the weight crept back on because I wasn't able to get down to the pool as often as I used to.

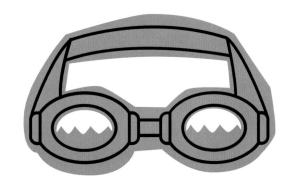

I also shifted my focus towards weights at the gym. If I'm honest, cardio exercise isn't my favourite thing... I am 6ft 3 and have a big build. I'm not made for running!

But recently I gave cycling a go – it turns out I enjoy it and I love being out in the fresh air. What I'm saying is you need to find whatever it is that makes you feel good, whether it's rock climbing, canoeing, martial arts or jogging round the park with your dog. Whatever it is – and there are so many options now – just find something that will stick.

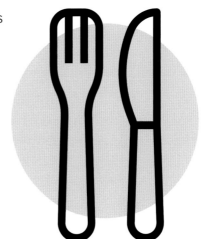

For fitness to be sustainable, you have to embrace it! It's easy to keep old bad habits going so you need to force yourself to make new healthy ones instead. I've now found a balance between gym, pool, cycling and eating healthy foods that seems to be working for me. It's all about creating new routines that will stick, and soon those positive choices that may seem so hard at first will become your new normal.

To get you started, my mate Adam, who is a personal trainer and fitness coach, has shared some easy but really effective exercises in the back of this book, as well as some top advice. The beauty of these moves is that they can be done anywhere, any time, and you can even break them into two parts if you like and do half in the morning, half at night. Or whatever works for you. They also cover cardio and strength in one go. It's a great way to kick-start your fitness, as you don't have to fork out for an expensive gym membership or allow for the added time to travel there and back. You can do Adam's workout in your back garden or even in your living room! This can really take the pressure off if you're a bit nervous about getting back into a fitness regime, or starting completely from scratch.

That said, don't be afraid of going to the gym! People seem to have a fear that it'll be full of fitness-wear models and tanned, ripped bodies. Honestly, mostly gyms are full of middle-aged men and women with a bit of weight to lose – just like me – who are trying to get a bit healthier. And how motivating is that?! Surrounding yourself with like-minded people is a great way to stay encouraged. If you don't fancy the gym, then get down to the local park with some friends or join an organised park workout. And make sure those around you know what you're doing so they can support you in your challenge.

Goals!

I've learned that achieving good health and fitness requires some big changes to your overall mindset. It's a lot to do with mental strength and committing to yourself. I know from experience that this is something you have to keep working hard at *all the time*. It's not easy! If it was, we'd all be walking around with six-packs. It's about identifying the reason why you want to lose weight in the first place – the bigger picture plan – and then to keep reminding yourself of that motivation when it gets tricky along the way, or when you hit a stumbling block. For me, it's Little Man, my son Acey – to be able to run about with him and, ultimately, to try and be around for him for as long as possible. And it's also about feeling healthier in myself; being able to climb a flight of stairs without getting out of breath.

Setting yourself some shorter-term goals is a fantastic way to kick-start your new routine and it can really help keep you focused and motivated – whether that's lifting another 10kg in the gym, finishing a certain distance in a quicker time, or swimming more laps of the pool in a single session. Mini-goals like this keep my workouts interesting, and my fitness and weight loss heading in the right direction.

It helps to set yourself a longer-term goal too, one that's clear and focused, rather than vague and general. This is called a 'SMART' goal, where SMART stands for Specific, Measurable, Attainable, Relevant and Timely. What this means is that your goal should be something that you can realistically achieve in a given time-frame. It should also be easy to measure so you can track your progress. So, losing a couple of stone to fit into your wedding gear next year is a great goal to aim for, or training so you can do a 10k run 3 months from now.

Be sure to choose a goal that you actually *want* to achieve so it will keep you motivated – there's no point in opting for something wildly unrealistic or that you don't really care about. Then break that goal down into some smaller milestones to tick off along the way.

No one is asking you to run 100 metres in 10 seconds or dead-lift 200kg. If you've not exercised in a long time – or ever – then even just taking a 10-minute walk is a great starting point, and you can build it up from there.

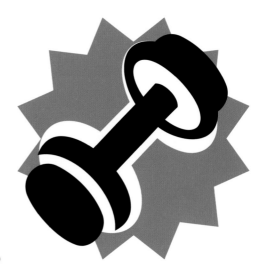

There are loads of tools to help you these days too, including apps to track what exercise you're doing and what you eat. It can be really surprising to learn how many calories some of your favourite foods actually contain, and once you become more aware of what you're eating by seeing it all written down, you'll hopefully be encouraged to make healthier choices. I love a gadget, so these apps have been hugely helpful for me, but my advice to you is not to become obsessed and also to be honest when you use them!

Fitness is great for setting goals: it's easy to see instant measurable results since it's all about the numbers – faster, longer, heavier... And when you hit those milestones, you'll notice that everything else in your life starts to feel easier too – walking to the shops, picking up the kids, just living every day with more energy.

If your alarm goes off at 6.30am and it's dark and cold outside and you think you can't face going for a run or doing your workout, remind yourself of your goals. Think back to how great it felt to achieve the latest milestone, imagine how amazing you are going to feel when you reach the next one and what it'll be like when you get to that final overall goal.

As you achieve each stage, take a moment to enjoy how great it feels! Once you experience that initial high of achievement, I promise you won't want to go back. Every new success will encourage you to work even harder and push for more. Just aim to be a little bit better every day. That's really all you can ask of yourself, and it's how I approach my business life too.

Another massive incentive is that you can find yourself starting to become an inspiration to other people too. Your children, partner, family, friends and colleagues will look at you and feel encouraged to live more healthily after seeing you make those changes in yourself. You will become other people's motivation, so don't let them down.

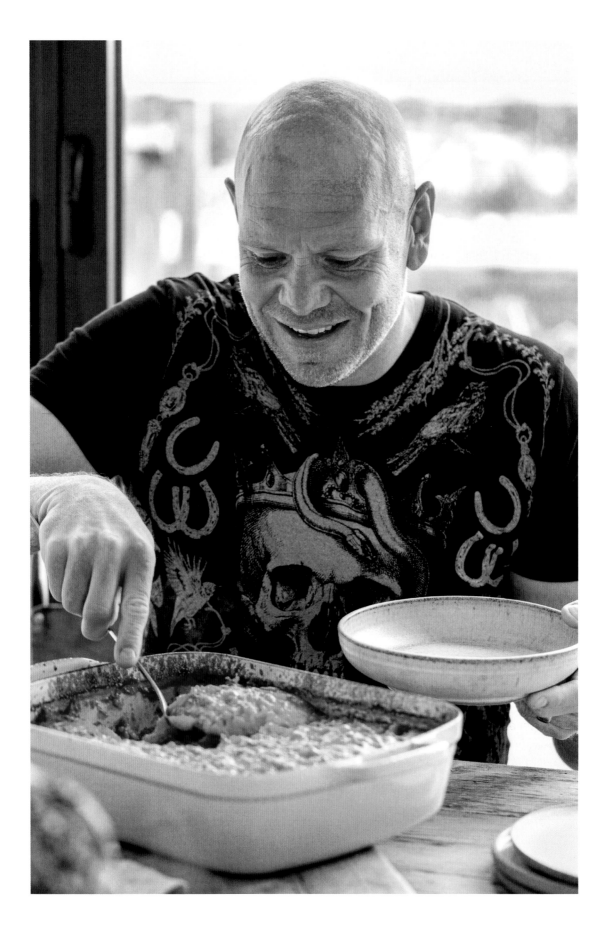

Enjoy your cooking

It goes without saying that I love food, I'm a professional chef after all! I am not about to start serving up bland, boring meals, even when I'm watching my weight. The number one rule when it comes to eating well on a diet is that you need to keep food interesting. It's so important to eat what you enjoy! This is about choice and being in control, so that your diet sticks long term. Everyone is different and has their own likes and dislikes, as well as different goals and different budgets – and maybe other family members to cater for.

I've made sure that every recipe in this book provides fantastic tastes and textures with each mouthful. They should also keep you feeling nice and full, since the portion sizes are generous. Eating a tiny plate of food would leave you hungry and disappointed – and more likely to fall off the wagon.

You'll see that I occasionally use reduced-fat and lower-calorie ingredients: 1-cal spray oil, reduced-fat dairy (yoghurt, soured cream, cheese or crème fraîche) and reduced-fat mayonnaise. However, many reduced-fat and low-calorie alternatives are lacking in flavour, and they can be full of sugars and other additives to make them taste better, so I'm more inclined to avoid them.

To achieve maximum flavour and texture I like to use a small amount of a high-calorie ingredient in a clever way. It could be a splash of full-fat coconut milk to add extra creaminess, or some smoked salmon, chorizo, cheese, nuts, chocolate or cocoa powder to boost the flavour. These are the kinds of ingredients that go a long way towards making your food taste substantial, giving your dishes a touch of unexpected luxury.

Spices, herbs, chilli and garlic are also brilliant ways of upping the flavour in lower-calorie meals. And I use a few other intensely flavoured ingredients now and then too: dried mushrooms, tahini, rose harissa, preserved lemons and liquid aminos are all great things to keep in your cupboards, as they'll provide big hits of instant flavour from very small quantities; they all work well with fish, chicken, meat or vegetables. Try the harissa salmon on page 148, the

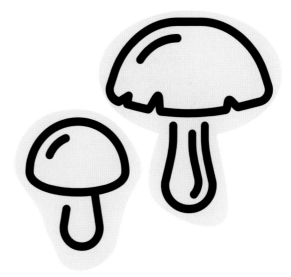

chicken, miso and mushroom ramen on page 174 or the saffron chicken burgers on page 164. And I use fresh stock when I can – either freshly made or from the supermarket chilled cabinet – it makes such a difference. It's absolutely fine to use a stock cube if you haven't got any fresh stock to hand, but avoid fish stock cubes as these tend to overpower the other flavours in a dish (use a vegetable stock cube instead).

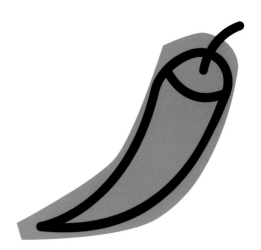

I also have a few other ways of adding extra flavour and texture without blowing the calories. It may sound a bit cheffy, but blow-torching meat and fish is easy and lends a lovely smoky taste and sticky, charred texture – the sort you get from roasting or frying in lots of fat. Roasting mince and toasting oats in the oven before you use them are other great ways to introduce more flavour – try the banana and pecan nut porridge on page 30 or the smoky beef chilli on page 197.

There's also a whole chapter devoted to sweet things, as I know this can be a particularly tough one for many dieters – from cakes to crumbles, there's something for everyone to enjoy. One thing I would say, though, is that as much as you shouldn't deprive yourself or say you can never eat your favourite snack ever again, I'm not a big fan of cheat days – I just think you're only cheating yourself.

In my experience, life tends to throw these days at us anyway. Maybe it's your anniversary and you're going out for dinner, or it's your best mate's birthday and they've made a decidedly non-diet chocolate cake. Or maybe you're stuck in traffic at dinner time and are forced to put a meal together at a roadside service station. There will always be moments like this that pop up from time to time, so don't worry about them when they do. If you're eating properly the rest of the time then you won't be derailing all your hard work – just get yourself back on track the next day. That said, you can put together a pretty healthy meal from a petrol station these days…

Get organised

Watching what you eat and making time to exercise is tough. Even if one week you're kicking it down at the gym and in the kitchen, there will be times when you'll waver. Trust me, I know the ups and downs well, and it's best to be prepared for them.

There are a few ways you can make it a bit easier and the most effective one is with a little bit of forward planning. Have a look through the recipes in this book and plan a few meals for the week – you can also turn to the Meal Prep chapter for some great pack-up-and-take-to-work lunch ideas to keep you going for a couple of days, like my teriyaki salmon or corn and black bean burrito bowls on pages 90 and 92. Most of my recipes are ready and on the table quickly so you don't have to spend hours cooking when you've got in from a heavy workout down the gym!

There are also lots of recipes that you can easily cook in a big batch then freeze what you don't eat straight away – look for the ❄ symbol. If you freeze meals in individual portions then you'll always have something healthy to hand that's ready to go when you need it. Remember to add a label so you know what it is later!

Don't be afraid to cut corners where you can either. I use some ready-cooked ingredients to speed things up – including pouches of cooked rice, lentils and quinoa, and roasted peppers in a jar. When you're in a rush they're the kind of convenience foods I fully support! If, however, you're cooking your own rice, lentils or quinoa, start with 60g per portion, which allows for the fact that the volume will more than double on cooking.

Get yourself some kitchen scales and a set of measuring spoons to keep quantities accurate. And a blender means you can whiz up soups, sauces and smoothies in seconds. It's also worth investing in some good storage containers, a thermal flask for soup and a drinks container for smoothies. That way you can take your meals with you, and you'll be less likely to give in to temptation when you're hungry.

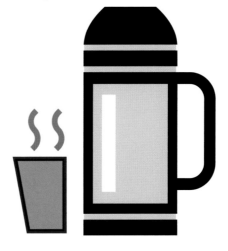

Lastly (*Rocky* theme plays)...

People sometimes worry that they're going to become boring or lose their personality if they start looking after themselves a bit more and change the way they eat. But remember that you're still *you*! In fact, in a way, you're even more *you* than you were before because you're now making decisions that are all about you. You're taking control of your life in a way you weren't before.

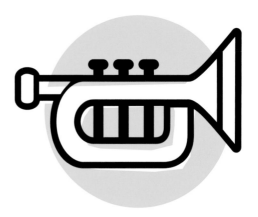

Sometimes I do miss those scrappy carefree days, when I ate and drank what I liked, and life was a bit more chaotic and spontaneous. But I wouldn't swap how I feel now to go back to who I was then. Never. I love waking up with a clear head and having so much more energy to put into my family, and as a chef and businessman. I have more clarity and focus in all areas of my life. I love feeling healthier and buying clothes that fit me more easily. And I definitely don't miss being out of breath just walking up a flight of stairs. It makes me happy knowing I'm looking after myself for me and my family. I did it, and now you can do it too.

THINGS TO REMEMBER

- Find a way to make your diet and new fitness targets work for you, otherwise you just won't stick to them.

- Set yourself achievable goals along the way, but always keep in mind the bigger picture of being fundamentally healthier and fitter.

- Time your workouts so they end at a mealtime: this way you won't be tempted to snack.

- But... always have a healthy snack to hand, just in case hunger takes you by surprise! Try hummus and carrots, or yoghurt and fruit.

- Learn to recognise whether you're actually hungry or not, and don't be afraid of a few hunger pangs.

- Be honest! If you're logging calorie intake or exercise on an app, you'll only be cheating yourself if you aren't truthful.

- Get into a competitive mindset where the sport is losing weight and getting healthy – and you want to win!

- But if you slip up, really don't beat yourself up about it, just think what you can do better next time.

- If you're heading out to eat, check out the food options before you go, so you don't get accidentally swayed into making an unhealthy choice.

- Enjoy it! Enjoy the wins, enjoy feeling healthier and enjoy taking positive control of your life.

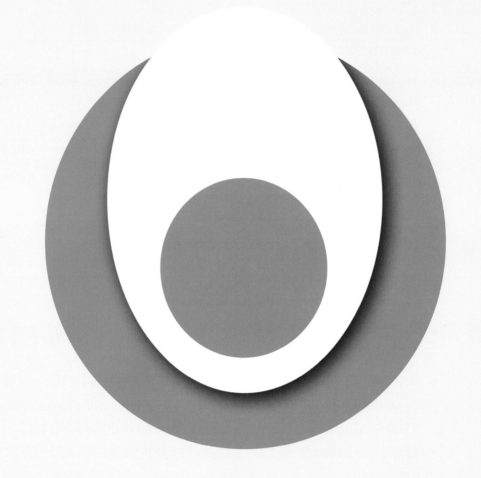

1 BREAKFAST

I NEVER USED TO BOTHER that much with breakfast – I'd just grab a quick coffee as I rushed out the door. But I've noticed that what I eat throughout the day makes a big difference to how I perform in my workouts, how I recover from them, and generally how much energy I have the rest of the time too. Eating properly first thing sets me up for the day and I now make a point of never skipping breakfast.

I usually get up really early to fit in some exercise before I head into work, so I'll often have some yoghurt and fruit before I go, and then take a pot of overnight oats with me to eat afterwards. These are so easy to prepare – they don't even involve any proper cooking! And you can add whatever flavours you like; try my peach Melba or apple and cardamom oats on pages 24 and 26. The breakfast muffins are also good to eat-on-the-go (see page 54) – make a batch and freeze them, then defrost one overnight for the morning.

This chapter is full of amazing ingredients that will power you through to lunchtime. I've used a lot of oats, which release their energy slowly and help you to refuel after a workout. Nuts are a brilliant addition too, as they are packed with healthy fats and protein. Scatter them over your porridge or have a go at making your own nut butter (see pages 48 and 50) to spread on toast for an instant breakfast. You'll find quite a few egg-based recipes too – eggs are incredibly versatile and a fantastic source of protein.

Breakfast is also a great opportunity to sneak in some extra fruit and veg. I've added broccoli to scrambled eggs (see page 36), rhubarb and banana to porridge (pages 29 and 30) and given avocado on toast an invigorating upgrade (page 47). When I have more time in the morning, the pancakes on page 53 are a surprisingly healthy option and fun to make with the kids.

Smoothies and shakes are another effective way to fuel up for the day and they're easy to whiz up in the morning. These shouldn't replace a proper meal, but I'll often have one before or after a workout to give me a bit of a boost if I need it. I've given some tasty combinations on pages 56–63, but feel free to try your own ideas, and get a portable drinks container so you can enjoy them on the move.

The recipes in this chapter are packed with healthy ingredients that are better for you than sugary cereals and will keep you feeling satisfied. They taste so much better too! I guarantee that if you make the effort to eat a delicious, filling breakfast, your road to weight loss and fitness will be that much easier to stick to.

PEACH MELBA OVERNIGHT OATS

With its perfect balance of peach sweetness and raspberry tartness, the classic peach Melba dessert has stood the test of time. This breakfast version has all the lovely tastes of summer in one healthy bowl. It's so easy to make – just leave the oats to soak overnight and then stir through the fruit in the morning. ♡

SERVES 1

60g porridge oats
½ tsp ground cinnamon
1 tsp granulated sweetener
60g tinned peaches (in natural juice), drained and roughly chopped, plus 2 tbsp juice from the tin
100ml whole milk
100g Greek yoghurt (0% fat)
A large handful (50g) raspberries
1 tbsp toasted flaked almonds
1 tsp honey

1 Place the porridge oats in a plastic container. Add the cinnamon and sweetener, stir to distribute, then add the peach juice, milk and yoghurt. Stir well until evenly mixed. Put a lid on the container and place in the fridge overnight.

2 The next morning take the overnight oats out of the fridge and stir in a little water to loosen the mixture. Stir in half of the peaches and raspberries and pour into a bowl.

3 Top with the remaining peaches and raspberries, scatter over the flaked almonds and trickle the honey over to serve.

Per serving: *534 cals*
26g protein   *66g carbs*
17g fat   *8g fibre*

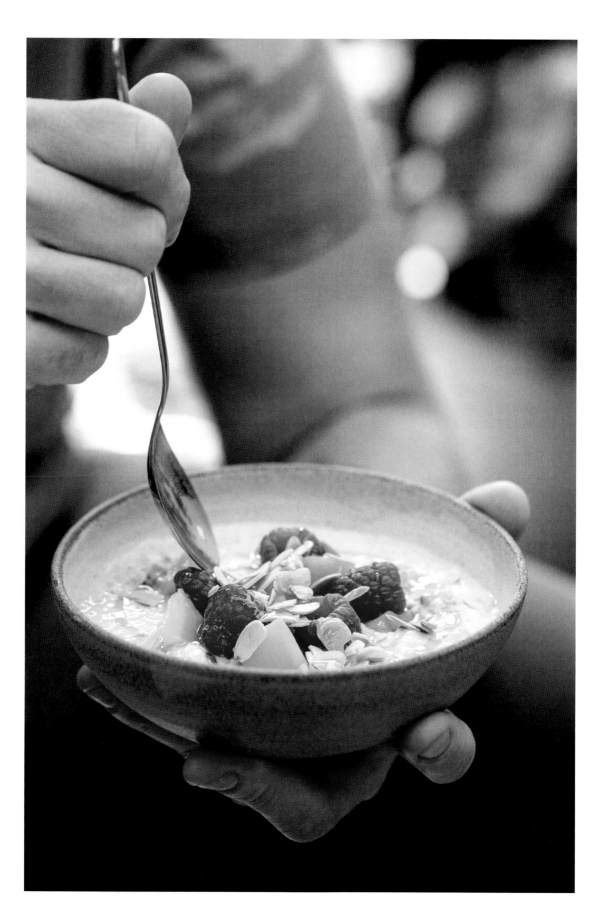

APPLE AND CARDAMOM OVERNIGHT OATS

This fruity oat pot couldn't be easier – you just soak the oats overnight and then add the apples the next day. The unexpected flavours of honey, apple, vanilla and cardamom turn a very simple recipe into an exciting and uplifting breakfast.

SERVES 1

60g porridge oats
50ml unsweetened apple juice
100ml whole milk
100g Greek yoghurt (0% fat)
¼ tsp ground cinnamon
1 tbsp granulated sweetener
15g raisins
1 tbsp honey
1 apple, peeled, cored and
   roughly chopped
½ tsp vanilla paste
A big pinch of ground
   cardamom
2 tbsp water

1 Place the porridge oats in a plastic container. Add the apple juice, milk, yoghurt, cinnamon, sweetener and raisins and stir well. Cover with a lid and place in the fridge overnight.

2 The next morning, place a small non-stick frying pan over a medium to high heat. When hot, add the honey, apple, vanilla paste, cardamom and water. Cook for 3–5 minutes, stirring occasionally. Remove from the heat.

3 Take the overnight oats out of the fridge and stir in a little water to loosen the mixture. Pour into a bowl and top with the apple mixture.

 BONUS Oats release their energy slowly, helping to sustain you for longer so you're less likely to feel the need for a snack mid-morning.

Per serving: 522 cals
22g protein   85g carbs
9g fat   6g fibre

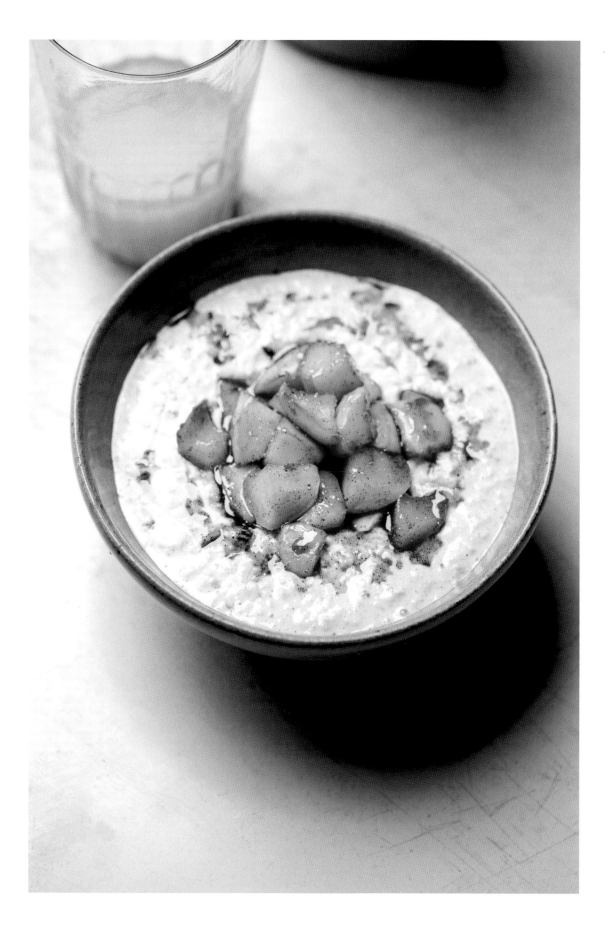

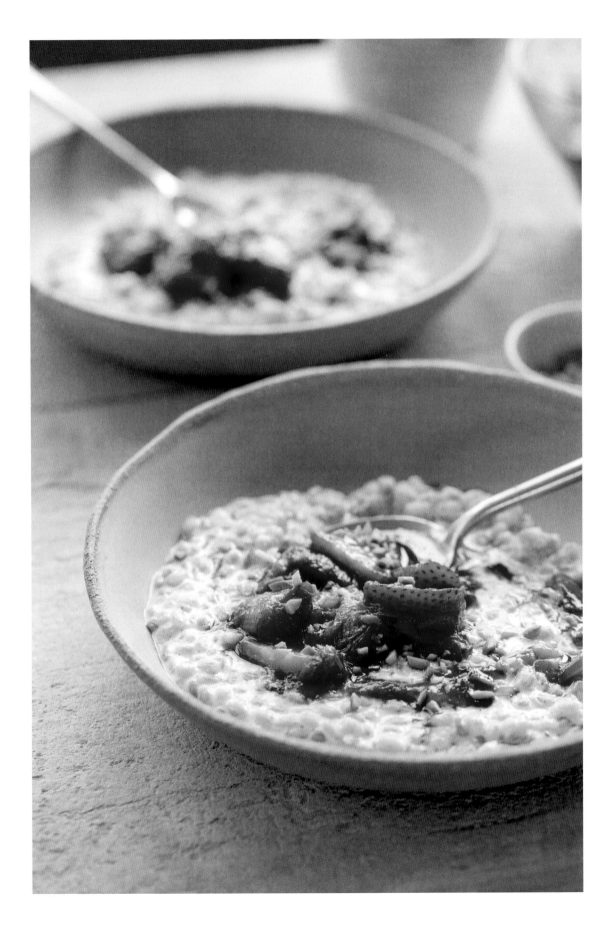

BARLEY PORRIDGE WITH RHUBARB COMPOTE

Using pearl barley instead of regular oats gives your morning porridge a different texture – it's a bit like a breakfast risotto! The rhubarb, ginger and citrus compote tastes amazing but feel free to use whatever fruit is in season, such as apples or pears. ♡

SERVES 2

120g pearl barley
500ml water
150ml whole milk
2–3 tsp granulated sweetener
A pinch of ground cinnamon
A pinch of sea salt
1 vanilla pod, split and seeds scraped
100ml single cream

For the rhubarb compote
200g rhubarb, cut into 2cm lengths
Finely grated zest of ½ orange
Juice of 1 orange
1 ball (20g) preserved stem ginger in syrup, finely chopped
1 tsp granulated sweetener
80g strawberries, thickly sliced

To serve
1 tbsp nibbed pistachio nuts

1 Put the pearl barley into a small saucepan and pour in the water. Place over a high heat and bring to the boil. Reduce the heat and simmer for 25 minutes or until the barley is just tender.

2 Meanwhile, make the compote. Place the rhubarb, orange zest and juice, stem ginger and sweetener in a small saucepan. Bring to a simmer over a medium heat, then cook for about 5 minutes until the rhubarb is just soft. Stir in the strawberries and remove from the heat.

3 Once the barley is tender, add the milk, sweetener, cinnamon, salt, vanilla seeds and cream to the pan. Stir well, increase the heat a little and cook for another 7–8 minutes or until the porridge is thick and creamy. If you prefer a looser consistency, stir in a little water.

4 Spoon the porridge into bowls and top with the compote and a sprinkle of pistachios for crunch.

Per serving: *477 cals*
12g protein   *65g carbs*
18g fat   *4g fibre*

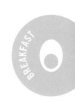

BANANA AND PECAN NUT PORRIDGE

Toasting the oats beforehand is a great way of enhancing the taste of this classic porridge recipe, while the banana and pecan topping adds extra layers of flavour and texture. ♡

SERVES 1

50g rolled oats
1 heaped tbsp pecan nuts
100ml whole milk
100ml water
1 banana, thickly sliced

1 Preheat the oven to 200°C/Fan 180°C/Gas 6.

2 Spread the oats out on a baking tray and toast in the oven for 10 minutes, until starting to turn golden brown and a little crunchy. On a separate tray, toast the pecans for 5 minutes.

3 Put the oats into a small saucepan and pour in the milk and water. Stir then bring to the boil over a medium heat. Lower the heat to a simmer and cook, stirring from time to time, for 4–5 minutes until the oats are tender.

4 Serve the porridge topped with the sliced banana and toasted pecans.

BONUS Nuts are packed with iron and healthy fats needed for post-exercise recovery, but if you are looking to cut down on the calories, leaving off the pecans will save you 106 cals.

Per serving: *457 cals*
12g protein   *58g carbs*
18g fat   *6g fibre*

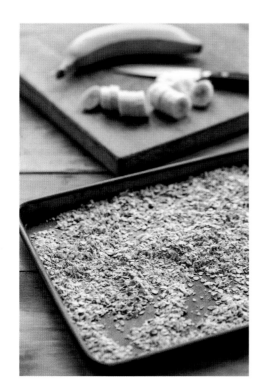

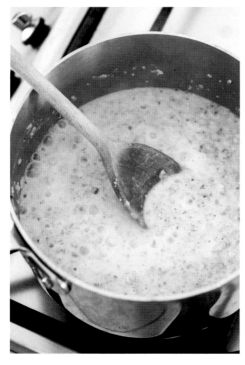

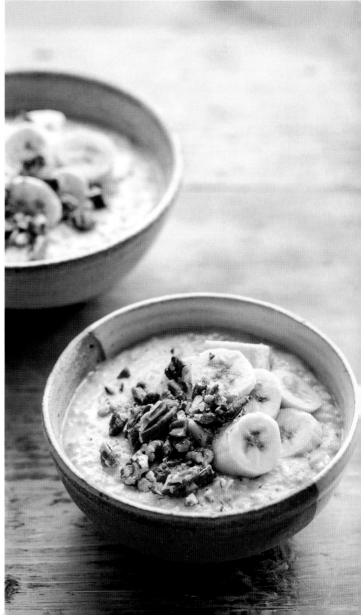

LADY GREY QUINOA PORRIDGE WITH BLUEBERRIES

Quinoa is a fashionable ingredient to use in salads now, but it is also a great alternative to oats when you're making porridge as it takes on other flavours well. Lady Grey tea and coconut is a lovely, subtle combination – Earl Grey will work too, it'll just be a bit stronger. The blueberry compote, with its hint of cardamom, gives a contrasting layer of fruity freshness. ♡

SERVES 2

150g white quinoa
2 Lady Grey tea bags
400ml water
100ml tinned coconut milk,
    plus a little extra to loosen
    if required
50ml single cream
2 tsp granulated sweetener

For the blueberry compote
175g blueberries
A pinch of ground cardamom
1 tbsp honey
1 tsp granulated sweetener
Juice of ½ lemon

To serve
2 tbsp flaked almonds, toasted

1 Rinse the quinoa in a sieve under cold running water and drain.

2 Put the quinoa into a small saucepan, add the tea bags and pour in the water. Bring to the boil over a medium heat then reduce the heat to a simmer and cook for 7–8 minutes. Remove the tea bags then add the coconut milk, cream and sweetener and cook for another 3–4 minutes or until the quinoa is tender. You can add a little more coconut milk for a looser consistency if you like.

3 For the compote, put all the ingredients into a small saucepan and bring to a simmer over a medium heat. Cook for 5 minutes or until the blueberries have burst and broken down slightly.

4 Serve the quinoa in bowls, topped with the blueberry compote and sprinkled with the toasted almonds.

BREAKFAST

Per serving: *471 cals*
14g protein   *55g carbs*
20g fat   *7g fibre*

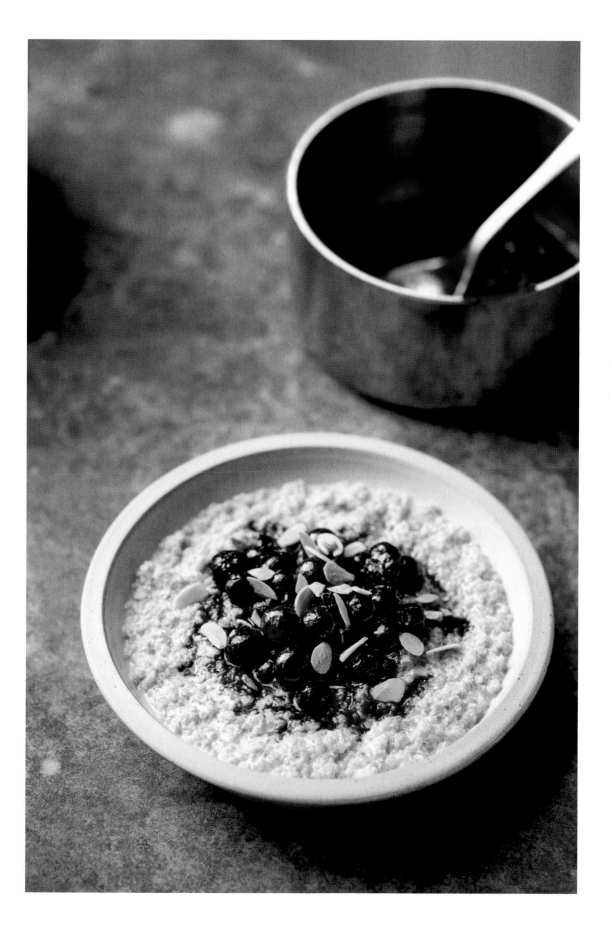

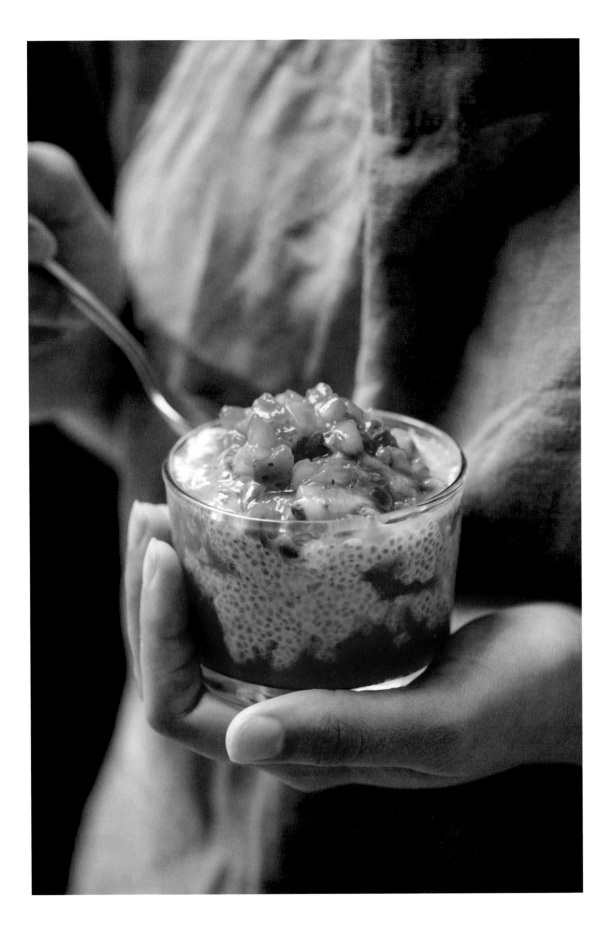

STRAWBERRY AND PASSION FRUIT CHIA POTS

Chia seeds lend an amazing, thick consistency to recipes and they are an excellent source of protein. The strawberry purée and passion fruit topping complement these vanilla-infused chia pots perfectly. A delicious way to start the day. ♡

SERVES 4

For the strawberry purée
200g strawberries, sliced
1 tbsp maple syrup
1 tsp granulated sweetener
1 tbsp water

For the chia pudding
120g chia seeds
1 vanilla pod, split and seeds scraped
3 tsp granulated sweetener
1 tbsp maple syrup
250ml whole milk
300g Greek yoghurt (0% fat)

For the topping
2–3 passion fruit, halved and pulp scooped out (50g prepared weight)
125g strawberries, finely chopped

1 Put the sliced strawberries, maple syrup, sweetener and water into a small saucepan and place over a medium heat. Bring to a simmer and cook gently for 5–7 minutes or until the strawberries are softened.

2 Transfer the mixture to a mini food processor and blend until smooth. Divide the strawberry purée between 4 serving glasses and leave to cool.

3 Meanwhile, to make the chia pudding, put the chia and vanilla seeds, sweetener, maple syrup, milk and yoghurt into a medium bowl and whisk together until evenly combined then leave to stand and thicken for 5 minutes.

4 Divide the chia mixture evenly between the serving dishes and place in the fridge. Leave overnight to set (see note).

5 Spoon the passion fruit pulp on top of the chilled chia puddings and pile the chopped strawberries on top to serve.

NOTE The chia puddings will be ready to eat after chilling for 30 minutes, but will still have a little bit of crunch. If you leave them in the fridge overnight they'll have a thicker and smoother texture.

Per serving: 268 cals
17g protein 19g carbs
11g fat 13g fibre

BREAKFAST

BROCCOLI, FETA AND DILL SCRAMBLED EGGS

Feta and dill are fantastic Greek flavours that remind me of my summer holidays. A splash of cream – although a bit of a luxury when you're on a diet – really lifts scrambled eggs, and tucking into this will feel like a decadent morning treat. ♡

SERVES 1

1-cal olive oil spray
100g tenderstem broccoli,
   trimmed and halved
1 tbsp water
2 large free-range eggs
1 tbsp dill, finely chopped
2 tbsp single cream
25g feta cheese, crumbled
½ red or green chilli, finely
   chopped
30g baby spinach
Sea salt and freshly ground
   black pepper

To serve
A handful of rocket leaves
   or salad cress
Lemon wedge

1 Place a medium non-stick frying pan over a medium heat. When hot, add a few sprays of oil followed by the broccoli and water. Cook for 2–3 minutes, tossing the broccoli every now and then.

2 Meanwhile, crack the eggs into a medium bowl and add the dill, cream, feta and chilli. Season with salt and pepper (you won't need much salt as the feta is already salty).

3 Add the spinach to the broccoli, season with salt and pepper and stir until the spinach begins to wilt.

4 Pour the egg mixture into the frying pan and cook for 1–2 minutes until the egg is just firm in some places but still a bit loose in others.

5 Slide the broccoli and scrambled egg mixture out of the pan onto a plate and serve with rocket leaves or salad cress, and a lemon wedge on the side.

 BONUS Eggs are a great, cheap source of healthy protein. I always have a stash of large free-range eggs in my fridge for quick scrambled eggs and omelettes.

Per serving: *326 cals*
25g protein   *4g carbs*
22g fat   *4g fibre*

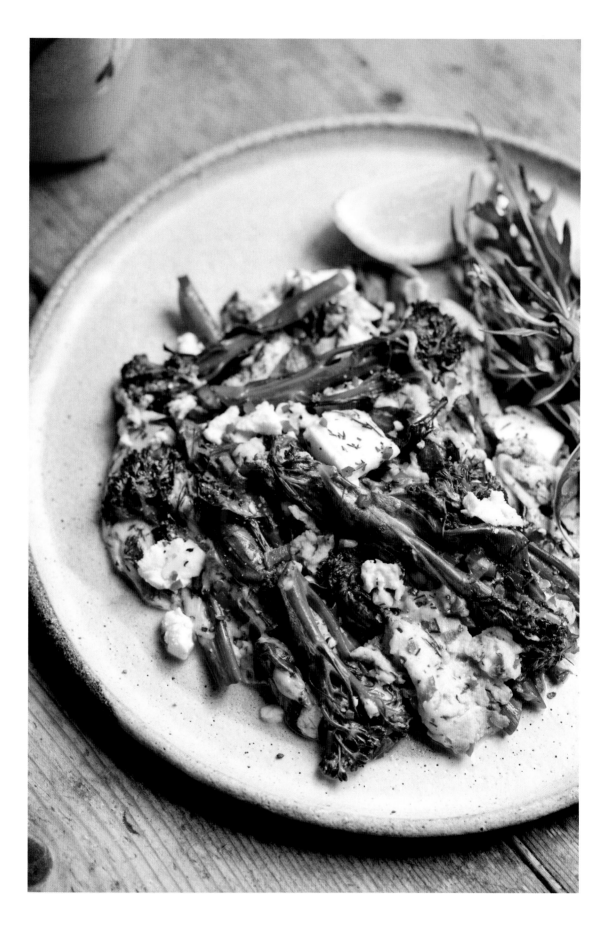

CHICKEN AND LEEK BAKED OMELETTE

You probably already know by now that I am really keen on tasty omelettes. Enriched with classic pie filling ingredients – chicken and leeks – this one combines two of my favourite things but without the added calories of pastry!

SERVES 4

2 tbsp light vegetable spread
2 leeks, finely sliced
2 garlic cloves, finely chopped
300g chicken breast, thinly sliced
½ chicken stock cube
2 tbsp finely chopped tarragon
2 handfuls (60g) baby spinach
4 large free-range eggs
50g ricotta cheese
50ml single cream
50g grated reduced-fat cheese
Sea salt and freshly ground black pepper
Mixed salad, to serve

1 Preheat the oven to 200°C/Fan 180°C/Gas 6 with the grill element on.

2 Melt half of the vegetable spread in a medium (25cm) ovenproof non-stick frying pan over a medium heat. Add the leeks along with a little seasoning and cook for 3–4 minutes. Add the garlic and cook for a further 2 minutes or until the leeks start to brown. Tip the leeks out onto a plate; return the pan to a high heat.

3 Add the remaining vegetable spread to the pan and once it is melted add the chicken. Crumble over the stock cube and cook for 3–4 minutes, stirring often, or until the chicken is cooked through.

4 Return the softened leeks to the pan and add the tarragon and spinach. Cook for 2 minutes or until the spinach has wilted.

5 In a bowl or jug, beat the eggs with the ricotta, cream and some seasoning. Pour the eggs into the pan and cook for a couple of minutes, without stirring.

6 Sprinkle the grated cheese over the eggs and place the pan under the grill for 4–5 minutes or until the cheese is melted and golden. Serve immediately, with a little side salad.

Per serving: *292 cals*
32g protein   *3g carbs*
16g fat   *3g fibre*

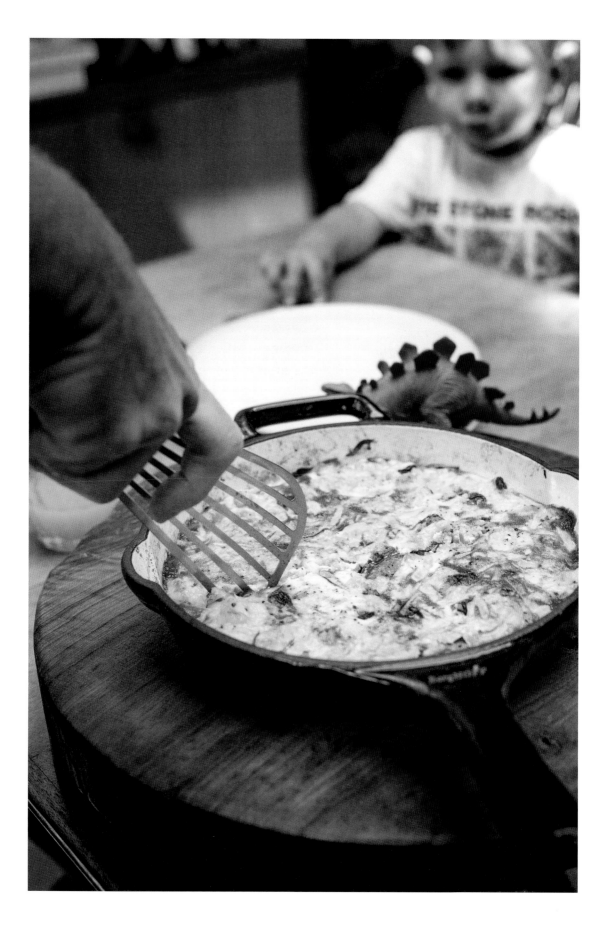

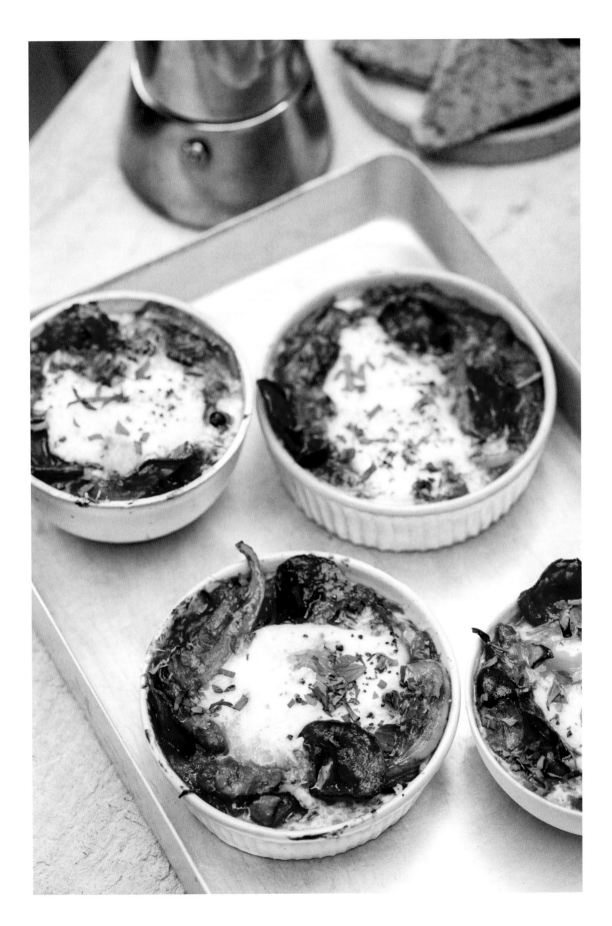

SPANISH-STYLE EGGS WITH CHORIZO

Chorizo isn't an ingredient you'd usually think about using when you're watching your weight but you only need a little bit to drive the flavours forward in this dish. Buy the spiciest chorizo you can get your hands on to give you more bang for your calorie buck!

SERVES 4

12 thin slices (40g) cooking chorizo sausage
1-cal olive oil spray
1 red onion, finely sliced
2 garlic cloves, thinly sliced
1 red pepper, cored, deseeded and thinly sliced
1 yellow pepper, cored, deseeded and thinly sliced
1 tsp sweet smoked paprika
2 tbsp tomato purée
2 x 400g tins chopped tomatoes
400g tin pinto beans or borlotti beans, drained and rinsed
50g pitted black olives, halved
50g baby spinach
4 large free-range eggs
15g Manchego cheese, finely grated
1 tbsp finely chopped flat-leaf parsley
Sea salt and freshly ground black pepper
4 slices wholegrain toast, to serve

Per serving: 393 cals
23g protein   39g carbs
13g fat   13g fibre

1 Preheat the oven to 200°C/Fan 180°C/Gas 6.

2 Place a large non-stick frying pan over a high heat. Add the chorizo slices and cook until crispy on both sides, then remove and drain on kitchen paper.

3 Place the pan back on the heat and spray a few times with oil. Add the onion and cook for 4–5 minutes until softened. Add the garlic and peppers and cook for a further 5 minutes or until the peppers are softened.

4 Stir in the paprika and cook for 1 minute, then stir in the tomato purée and cook for 2 minutes. Add the chopped tomatoes, pinto beans and black olives. Stir well and bring to a simmer, stirring occasionally. Cook for 10 minutes or until slightly thickened.

5 Stir in the spinach, cook briefly until just wilted and season with salt and pepper to taste.

6 Divide the mixture between 4 ovenproof dishes and stand them on a baking tray. Create a little well in the middle of each one, crack in an egg and sprinkle it with salt and pepper and a little grated cheese.

7 Bake in the oven for 5 minutes then take out the tray and tuck 3 slices of crispy chorizo into the sauce around each egg. Bake for a further 5–7 minutes or until the white of the egg is cooked completely and the yolk is soft. Sprinkle with the chopped parsley and serve at once, with wholegrain toast.

SALMON AND AVOCADO EGG-WHITE OMELETTE

POST

I love using hot-smoked salmon in cooking as it's high in flavour, has a great flaky texture and isn't quite as rich as regular smoked salmon. The lighter quality of egg-white omelettes is appealing in the morning. You can make this with whole eggs if you prefer, but you'll need to allow an extra 110 calories for the yolks.

SERVES 1

2 large free-range egg whites
　(80g)
1 tbsp finely chopped chives
1 tbsp finely chopped basil
1-cal olive oil spray
A large handful (30g) baby
　spinach, finely chopped
60g hot-smoked salmon (at
　room temperature), flaked
¼ ripe avocado, sliced
2 tbsp salad cress
Sea salt and freshly ground
　black pepper

1 In a medium bowl, whisk the egg whites, chives and basil together with some salt and pepper, until light and fluffy.

2 Heat a medium non-stick frying pan over a medium heat. When it is hot, add a few sprays of oil and pour in the egg white mixture, swirling the pan around so that the egg white reaches the edges evenly. Cook for 1 minute on one side then, using a fish slice, flip it over and cook for a minute on the other side. Slide the omelette out onto a warmed serving plate.

3 Put the pan back on the heat and spray a couple more times with oil. Add the spinach along with a little seasoning and stir until wilted.

4 Place the spinach on one half of the omelette and top with the salmon, avocado and most of the cress. Add a little more seasoning then fold the other side of the omelette over the filling. Serve at once, topped with the remaining cress.

Per serving:　*234 cals*
26g protein　*2g carbs*
13g fat　*2g fibre*

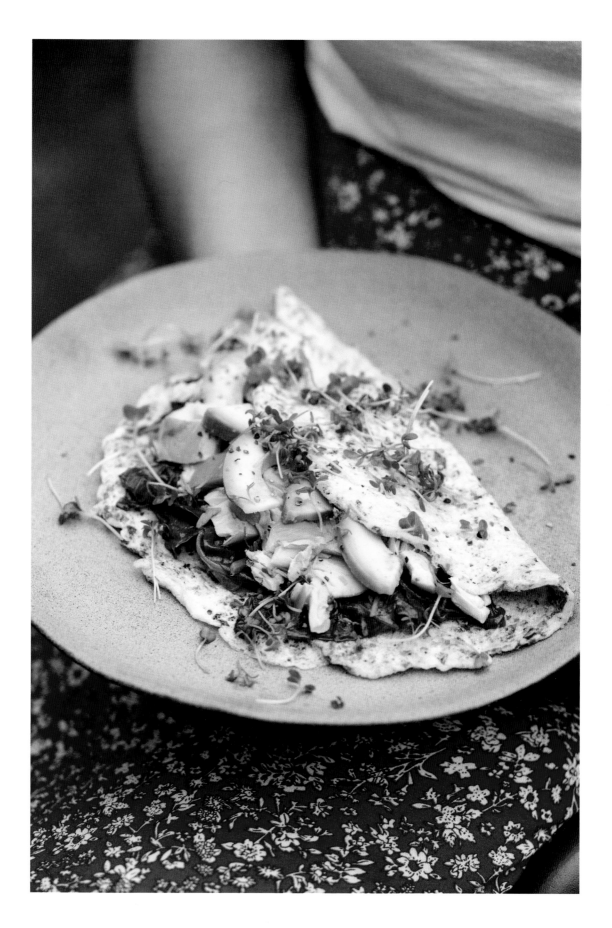

GREEN EGGS AND HAM

I'm a huge fan of kale – I love its big, strong, irony flavours and it works so well here with the sweetness of the peas and spring onions. If you can't get hold of ham hock, just use chopped-up sliced ham instead.

SERVES 2

100g flaked ham hock
4 large free-range eggs
50ml single cream
1 tbsp light vegetable spread
4 spring onions, finely sliced
2 garlic cloves, finely chopped
A large handful (50g) kale, finely chopped
A large handful (50g) baby spinach, finely chopped
80g frozen peas
Sea salt and freshly ground black pepper
2 slices wholegrain toast, to serve
1 tbsp (5g) finely grated Parmesan, to finish

1   Preheat the oven to 220°C/Fan 200°C/Gas 7. Line a baking tray with a silicone mat or baking paper.

2   Place the ham hock on the lined tray and cook for 12–15 minutes until crispy.

3   In the meantime, put the eggs, cream and a good pinch each of salt and pepper into a medium bowl and whisk together.

4   Melt the vegetable spread in a medium non-stick frying pan over a high heat. Add the spring onions and garlic and cook, stirring well, for 2–3 minutes.

5   Add the kale to the pan and cook for 2 minutes then stir in the spinach and peas. Season with a little salt and pepper and pour in the eggs. Leave them to set for a few seconds, then stir around in the pan to scramble for 1–2 minutes, until just firm in places but still loose in others.

6   Pile the scrambled eggs and greens onto the warm toast and sprinkle with the crispy ham hock and grated Parmesan to serve.

Per serving: *410 cals*
34g protein   *14g carbs*
23g fat   *5g fibre*

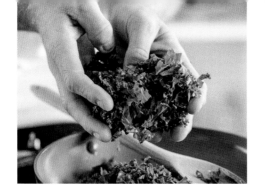

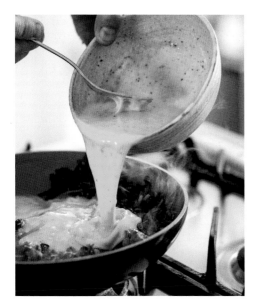

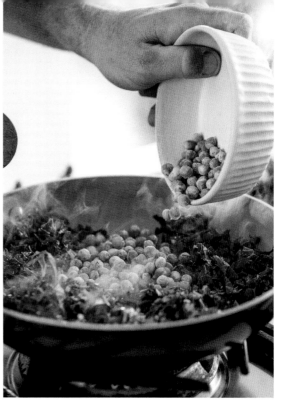

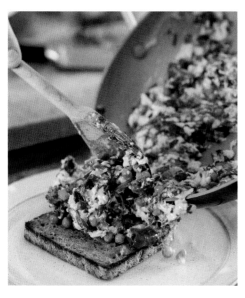

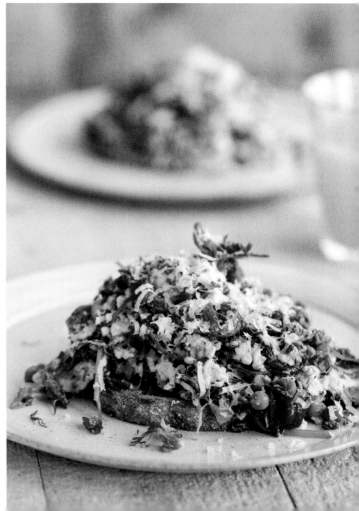

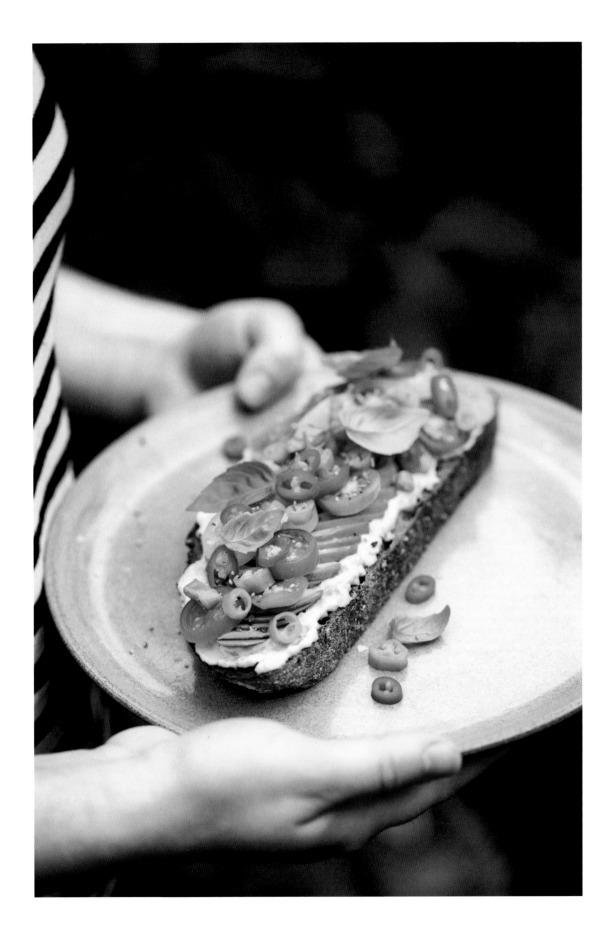

CHILLI AVOCADO TOAST

We all know that avocado on toast is one of the most popular breakfasts – it's been around for some years now – but adding a layer of hummus and spiking it with some chilli will turn it up a notch. Enjoy! ♡

SERVES 2

2 large slices wholemeal or
    brown sourdough bread
2 tbsp hummus
1 ripe avocado
80g cherry tomatoes, thickly
    sliced
4 pickled chillies or peppadew
    peppers, thinly sliced
1 red chilli, thinly sliced
A small handful of basil leaves
½ lime
Sea salt and freshly ground
    black pepper
Togarashi or dried chilli flakes,
    to sprinkle (optional)

1 Toast the sourdough bread and spread thickly with the hummus.

2 Halve the avocado, remove the stone and gently loosen the skin away from the flesh, using a large spoon. Thinly slice each avocado half, gently flatten with the palm of your hand and lift onto the toast.

3 Sprinkle with salt and pepper and top with the cherry tomatoes, pickled chillies, red chilli and basil leaves.

4 Squeeze over the juice from the lime half and serve at once, sprinkled with a little togarashi or chilli flakes if you like.

BONUS Avocados are loaded with heart-healthy fats. Don't be afraid of eating fats when you're on a diet, they help you feel full. Just limit your intake – of saturated fats in particular – and try to avoid fatty processed foods.

Per serving: *367 cals*
7g protein   *29g carbs*
23g fat   *7g fibre*

CRUNCHY NUT BUTTER

With its great balance of toasted nuts and a touch of sweetness from maple syrup, this nut butter tastes fantastic. Try the delicious pecan nut and cashew variations too, and experiment to find your own preferred nuts and flavouring combo. Allow 15g nut butter per serving for your calorie count. ♥

MAKES A 250g JAR

100g walnuts
100g pecan nuts
100g blanched hazelnuts
  (skinned)
A large pinch of flaky sea salt
1 tbsp maple syrup

1 Preheat the oven to 200°C/Fan 180°C/Gas 6.

2 Place the nuts on a baking tray and roast in the oven for 8–10 minutes. Remove and leave to cool slightly.

3 Put the nuts into a food processor and pulse briefly to chop finely. Take out a couple of spoonfuls and set aside on a plate.

4 Add the salt and maple syrup to the chopped nuts in the processor and blend again for another 10 minutes or until the nut butter reaches a creamy consistency. It may seize slightly, but just keep blending and it will come good (don't be tempted to add water, oil or anything else).

5 Scrape the mixture into a bowl and fold through the reserved chopped nuts.

6 Transfer the nut butter to a sterilised jar (see note on page 50), seal with a lid and label. Refrigerate and use within a month.

VARIATIONS

Pecan nut and honey butter: Use 300g pecan nuts (unsalted), a large pinch of flaky sea salt and 1 tbsp honey (instead of maple syrup).

Cashew and cardamom butter: Use 300g cashew nuts (unroasted and unsalted), a large pinch of flaky sea salt and 1 tbsp agave (instead of maple syrup), adding ½ tsp ground cardamom with the salt.

Per serving: *101 cals*
2g protein   *1g carbs*
10g fat   *1g fibre*

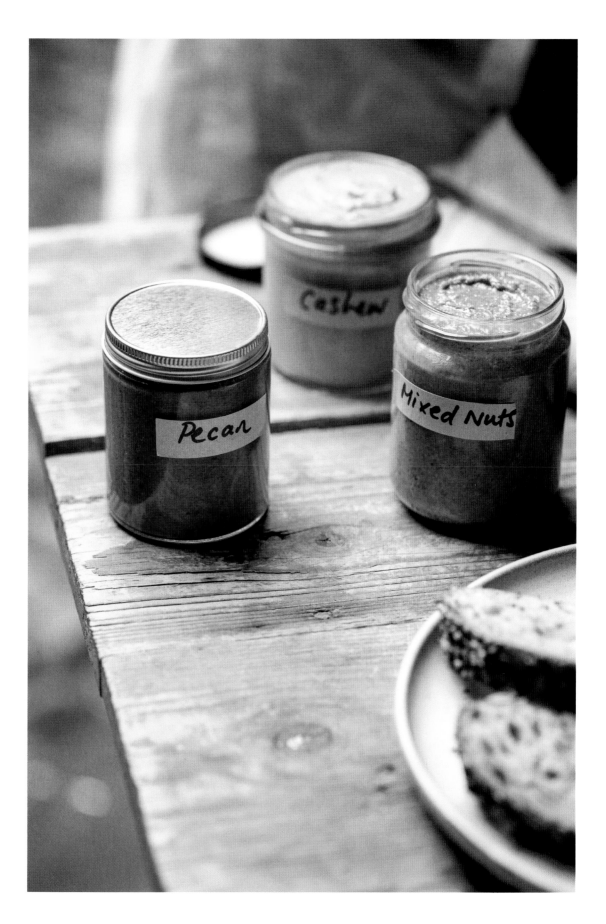

CHOCOLATE HAZELNUT SPREAD

I love chocolate spread, and making your own means you can control exactly what goes into it. The quality of the ingredients will really make a difference here, so buy the best cocoa powder you can find – and include that pinch of salt. Spread a bit on toast, skip the butter, and remember that a little goes a long way. Allow 15g per serving for your calorie count. ♥

MAKES A 450g JAR

200g blanched hazelnuts
(skinned)
80g good-quality cocoa powder
2 tbsp vanilla extract
50ml maple syrup
1½ tbsp granulated sweetener
200ml whole milk
A pinch of flaky sea salt

1 Preheat the oven to 200°C/Fan 180°C/Gas 6.

2 Spread the hazelnuts out on a baking tray and roast in the oven for 8 minutes or until they turn a deep golden brown. Remove and leave to cool slightly.

3 Put all the rest of the ingredients into a food processor, add the roasted hazelnuts and blend until smooth.

4 Transfer to a sterilised jar, seal with a lid and label. Refrigerate and use within a month.

VARIATION Use coconut or almond milk instead of cow's milk.

NOTE To sterilise jars, wash in hot soapy water, rinse well, then place upside down on a baking tray in a preheated oven at 120°C/Fan 100°C/Gas ½ to dry, or put them through a hot dishwasher cycle.

Per serving: *54 cals*
2g protein   *2g carbs*
4g fat   *1g fibre*

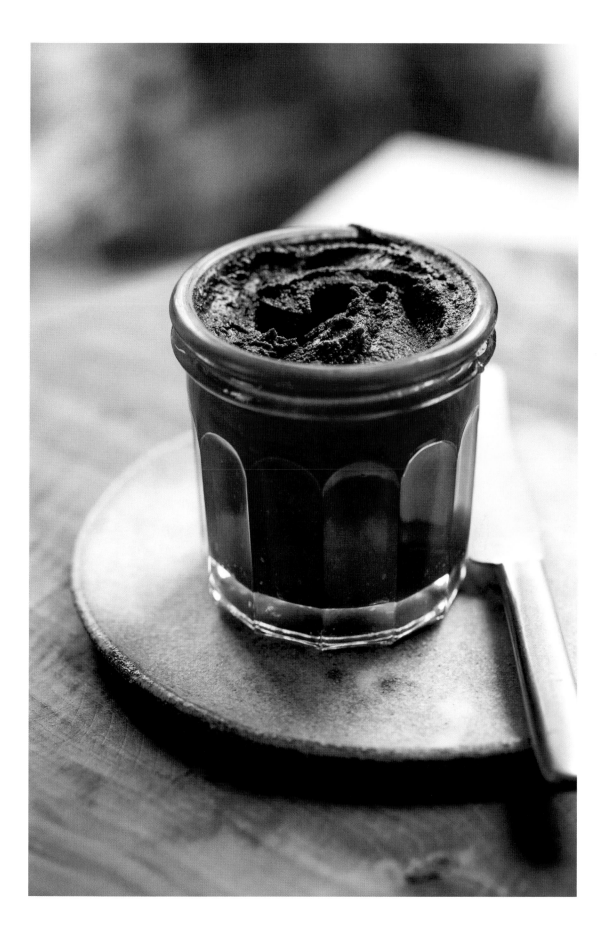

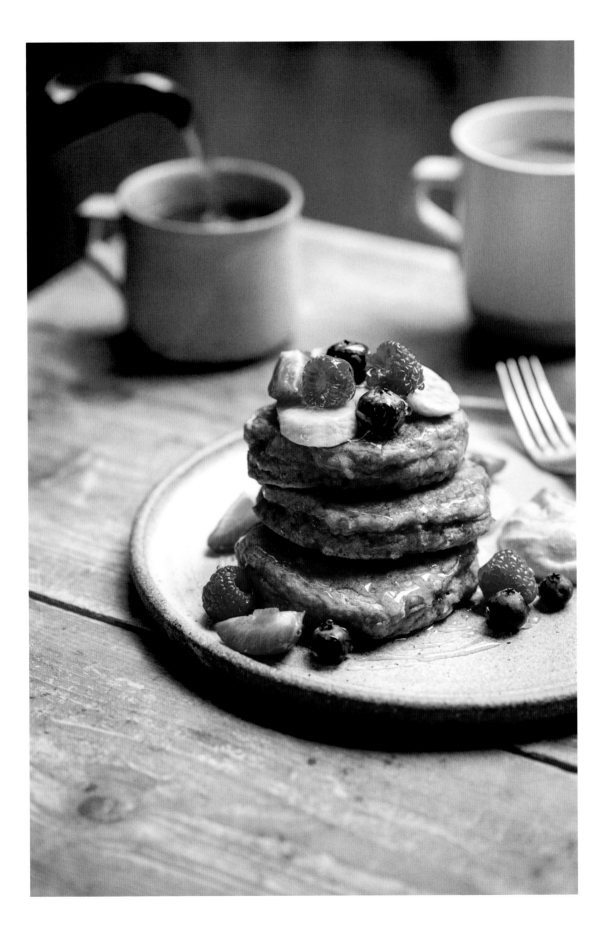

TAHINI AND HONEY PANCAKES

Pancakes are great to make with the family at weekends. They are often seen as a naughty treat, but wholemeal flour makes these a much healthier option. With its intense sesame flavour, tahini works well with the banana, cinnamon and cardamom. ⩔

SERVES 4

275ml whole milk
2 chai tea bags
½ tsp ground cinnamon
¼ tsp ground cardamom
250g self-raising wholemeal flour
1 tsp bicarbonate of soda
1 tsp cream of tartar
1 tsp granulated sweetener
2 tbsp tahini (35g)
125g banana, mashed
1 large free-range egg
1-cal sunflower oil spray

For the tahini yoghurt
100g Greek yoghurt (0% fat)
1 tbsp tahini
½ tsp granulated sweetener

For the topping
2 bananas, sliced
300g mixed berries (such as blueberries, raspberries and quartered strawberries)
4 tbsp honey

Per serving: 525 cals
20g protein   80g carbs
12g fat   11g fibre

1 Preheat the oven to 140°C/Fan 120°C/Gas 1.

2 To make the pancakes, pour the milk into a small saucepan. Cut open the tea bags and add the leaves to the milk, along with the cinnamon and cardamom. Bring to a gentle simmer over a medium heat, then remove from the heat and leave to cool slightly.

3 Stir the dry ingredients together in a large bowl. Put the tahini, banana and egg into a separate bowl and pour the tea-infused milk through a strainer over them. Whisk well to combine.

4 Pour the wet mix into the dry mixture and whisk well until combined, making sure there are no lumps.

5 Place two large non-stick frying pans over a medium heat and add a few sprays of oil to each. Drop 3 large spoonfuls of batter into each pan, spacing them well apart. Cook for 1 minute then flip each one over and cook on the other side for 1 minute; flatten them a little with the back of the spoon as they cook.

6 Place the 6 pancakes on a tray and keep warm in the oven, while you cook the second batch. For the tahini yoghurt, mix the ingredients together in a small bowl.

7 Pile the pancakes onto plates and top with the sliced bananas and berries. Add a drizzle of honey and serve with a dollop of tahini yoghurt.

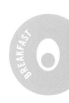

BREAKFAST MUFFINS

These are fun to make with the kids and are great for refuelling after a morning workout, or for eating on the go. The banana keeps the muffins moist and adds natural sweetness. Blueberries are great here, but feel free to use other berries if you like. ♡ ❄

MAKES ABOUT 12

100g rolled oats
120g self-raising wholemeal
    flour
2 tsp baking powder
1 tsp ground mixed spice
1 tsp ground cinnamon
250g Greek yoghurt (0% fat)
120ml whole milk
50g reduced-fat butter
    alternative, melted
3 large free-range eggs,
    lightly beaten
2 tbsp vanilla extract
4 tbsp granulated sweetener
300g bananas (about 2 large),
    mashed
150g fresh blueberries

For the topping
30g mixed seeds
1 tbsp rolled oats
1 tbsp demerara sugar

1 Preheat the oven to 200°C/Fan 180°C/Gas 6. Have ready a 12-hole silicone muffin tray if you have one, or line a standard muffin tray with silicone or paper muffin cases.

2 Tip the oats into a food processor and blitz to the consistency of flour. Add all the remaining ingredients, except the mashed bananas and blueberries, and blend until smooth.

3 Transfer the mixture to a large bowl and fold through the mashed bananas and blueberries. Spoon the mixture evenly into the muffin cases.

4 For the topping, mix the seeds, oats and sugar together. Sprinkle over the tops of the muffins.

5 Bake in the oven for 20–25 minutes or until the muffins are risen, golden and cooked through. Transfer to a wire rack and allow to cool a little. Eat while still warm if you can!

TO FREEZE Allow to cool, then freeze in ziplock bags or a rigid container. Defrost at room temperature any time you need a quick breakfast or treat. You can also reheat the muffins in an oven preheated to 180°C/Fan 160°C/Gas 4 for 5 minutes.

Per muffin: 175 cals
8g protein   22g carbs
6g fat   3g fibre

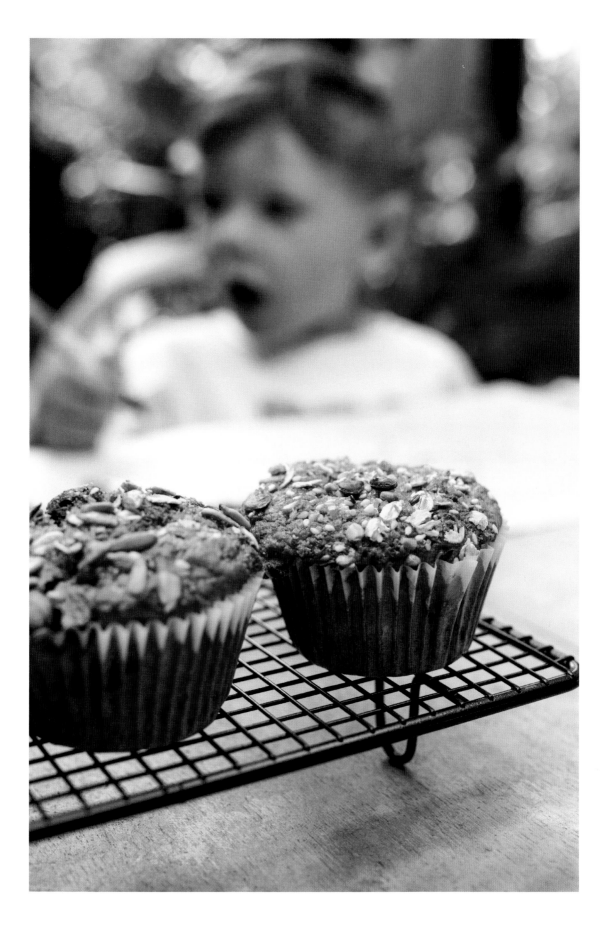

NUTTY BANANA BREAKFAST SHAKE

This is a great quick breakfast for those mornings when you're in a rush – stick it in a drinks container and have it on the way to work. It's a bit like a blended porridge, with the flavours of banana, cinnamon and vanilla working together beautifully. You can also go the extra mile and use homemade nut butter (see page 48). ∨

 POST

SERVES 1

180ml whole milk
20g porridge oats
1 tbsp nut butter
1½ bananas, peeled and
    frozen in a ziplock bag
1 tsp granulated sweetener
1 tsp vanilla extract
A pinch of ground cinnamon
2–3 ice cubes

1 Put all the ingredients into a jug blender and blend until completely smooth.

2 Pour into a large glass or portable drinks container and enjoy!

VARIATION Use coconut or almond milk instead of cow's milk.

 BONUS To lower the calorie count, simply leave out the nut butter – this will save you 101 calories. The shake will still be satisfying and delicious.

Per serving: *424 cals*
12g protein   *52g carbs*
18g fat   *5g fibre*

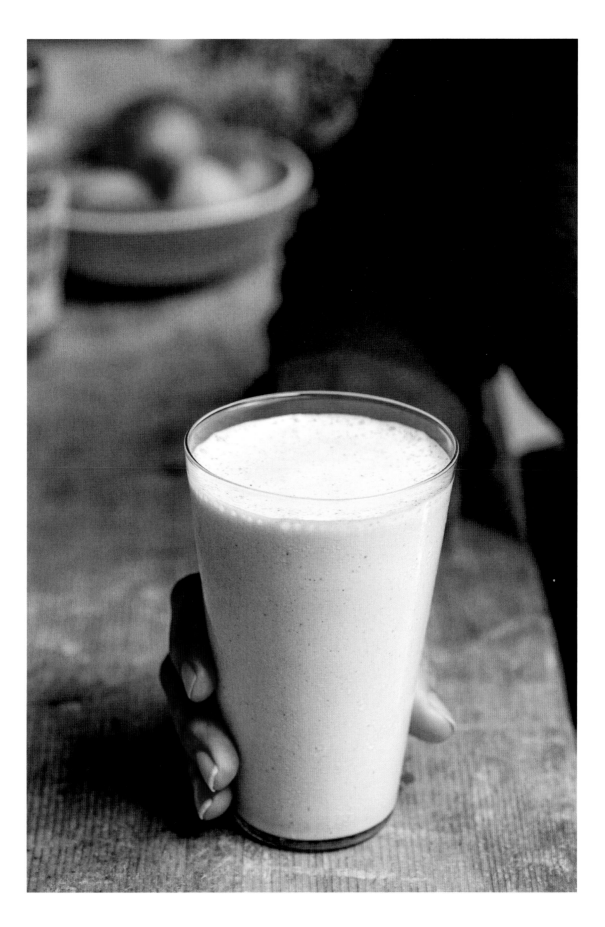

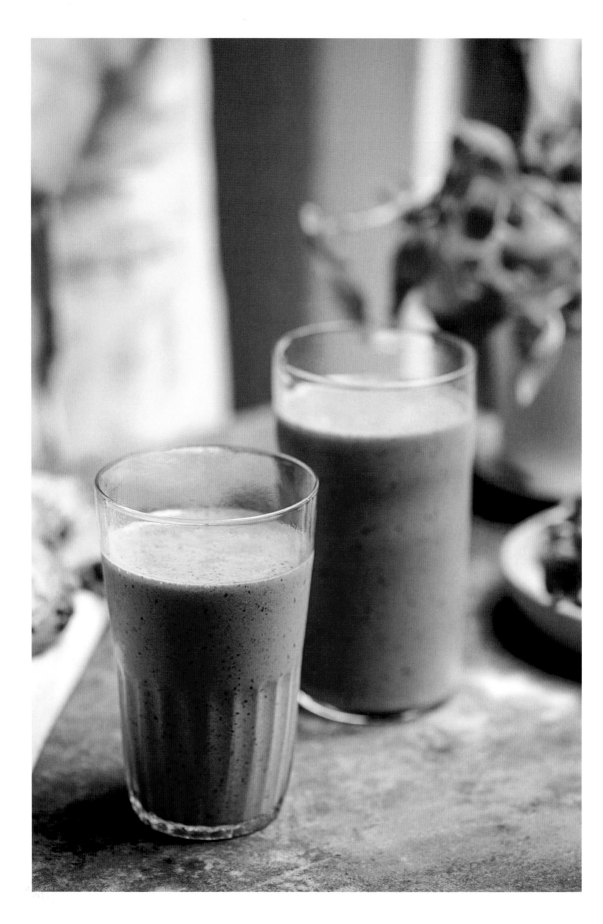

BERRY AND YOGHURT BREAKFAST SHAKE

I'll often have this shake when I want to refuel after morning exercise. By keeping a stash of berries in the freezer I can whiz it up in seconds, and avoid giving in to hunger cravings on the way back from the gym. ♡

SERVES 1

A large handful (100g) frozen berries
30g porridge oats
2 tbsp Greek yoghurt (0% fat)
1 tsp granulated sweetener
180ml whole milk
A few mint leaves
4 ice cubes

1 Put all the ingredients into a jug blender and blend until completely smooth.

2 Pour into a large glass or portable drinks container and enjoy!

VARIATION Use coconut or almond milk instead of cow's milk.

BONUS This shake is ideal as a pre- or post-workout breakfast – the oats supply sustained energy while yoghurt provides protein to promote muscle recovery. And berries are a great source of vitamin C, which is also needed for muscle repair and helps to boost the immune system.

Per serving: *341 cals*
21g protein   *42g carbs*
9g fat   *6g fibre*

MOCHA 'GET UP AND GO' SHAKE

This is a proper wake-up shake to kick-start your morning and get you powered up for the day. The oats and banana will keep you going, and the shake has a welcome caffeine kick from the espresso. The addition of cocoa makes it feel a bit more special than your regular smoothie. ♥

SERVES 1

1 banana, peeled and
   frozen in a ziplock bag
2 tbsp good-quality cocoa
   powder
200ml whole milk
20g porridge oats
30ml shot of espresso or 1 tsp
   instant coffee granules
3–4 ice cubes

1 Put all the ingredients into a jug blender and blend until completely smooth.

2 Pour into a large glass or portable drinks container and enjoy!

VARIATION Use coconut or almond milk instead of cow's milk.

Per serving: *402 cals*
17g protein   *45g carbs*
15g fat   *8g fibre*

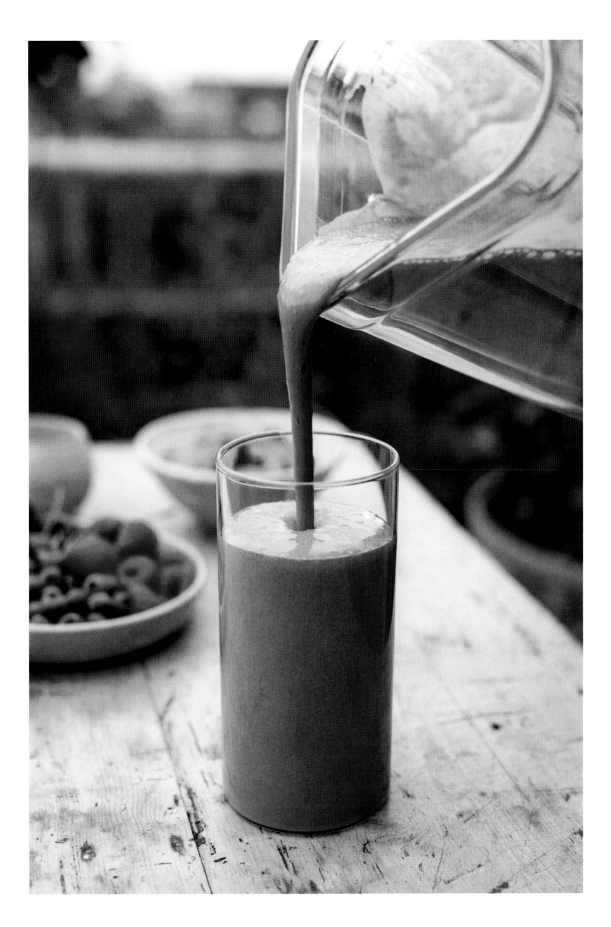

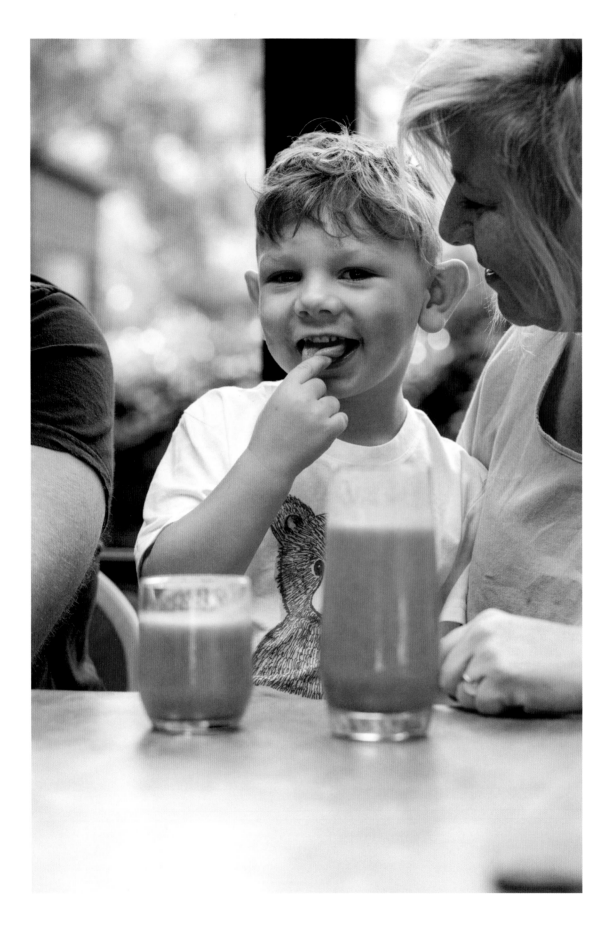

'GET YOUR GREENS IN' SMOOTHIE

Green smoothies are such an amazing way to start the day. You instantly know that you're doing your body some good – just look at that incredible colour! This one has a lovely natural sweetness from the pineapple, and the mint gives it a refreshing lift. ♡

SERVES 1

150ml unsweetened apple juice
150ml coconut water
A large handful (50g) baby spinach
A large handful (150g) frozen pineapple chunks
A small handful of mint leaves
½ ripe avocado, peeled
A small handful of ice cubes

1 Put all the ingredients into a jug blender and blend until completely smooth.

2 Pour into a large glass or portable drinks container and enjoy!

Per serving: *319 cals*
4g protein   *38g carbs*
15g fat   *6g fibre*

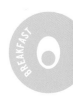

BREAKFAST

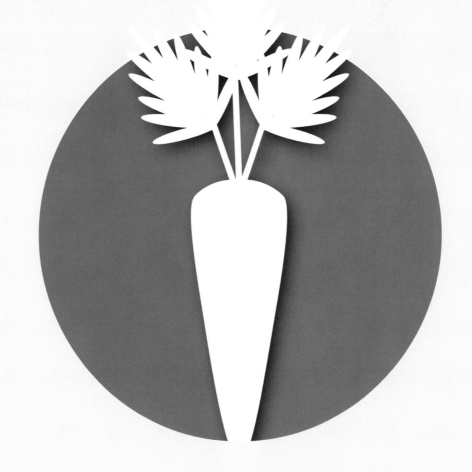

2 LIGHTER DISHES

IF YOU ARE FITTING IN A WORKOUT in the evening and don't fancy anything too heavy to eat for dinner, or maybe you've had a bigger meal at lunchtime, then this is the chapter for you. Most of these recipes are a bit lower in calories, and they also make use of fresher, lighter ingredients.

Fresh herbs, chillies and spices are all brilliant ways to introduce flavour to your cooking, while keeping calories low. I've packed fresh Thai basil, coriander and mint leaves into the prawn and avocado rice paper rolls on page 79, which are also perfect for taking to work in a lunchbox – don't forget to put the sauces in little pots for dipping!

Chickpeas, lentils and quinoa are great store-cupboard ingredients. They are amazing sources of meat-free protein, and if you buy some that are pre-cooked, you'll be able to make a tasty meal in minutes. I've really got into quinoa, as it takes on other flavours well; try it in the carrot and quinoa fritters or cauliflower quinoa couscous on pages 71 and 82. Lentils can also make a good low-fat alternative to meat. I've used them as a protein boost in the chicken and spinach samosas on page 76, which are baked in the oven rather than deep-fried, making them a healthier option.

Packs of prawns, feta and cooked beetroot are other healthy convenience foods that enable you to put together a delicious, nutritious plate of food with hardly any effort. Items like this all add a luxurious feel to mealtimes, so it won't seem like you're eating traditional 'diet food': I think this is the key to making healthy eating a part of your everyday life.

Frozen edamame beans stashed in the freezer are also useful for an extra protein and vitamin hit. I've used them in an Asian-style rice salad to go with the sticky chicken skewers on page 85, and they make an appearance in the beetroot and farro salad on page 66, which has the added bonus of being thrown together in under 20 minutes.

Some of these recipes can be made ahead, which really helps if you're squeezing in a workout and are a bit pushed for time. The smoked mackerel pâté and chickpea Scotch eggs on pages 68 and 72 will keep in the fridge for a couple of days, so you can have something tasty ready for you when you get home.

When you're watching your weight, you need to make every calorie count. The recipes in this chapter may be a bit lighter, but they are sky high in nutrients and flavour.

BEETROOT FARRO SALAD

Not many people cook with farro but it's a brilliant flavour vehicle, like quinoa and freekeh. Super-quick to put together, this combination of earthy beetroot and kale with creamy feta will make you feel like you've eaten so much more – which I know is key when you're on a diet! ♡

 POST

SERVES 2

100g quick-cook farro
100g frozen edamame beans
1 tbsp Dijon mustard
Juice of 2 lemons
2 tbsp extra-virgin olive oil
50g kale, tough stalks
    removed, roughly chopped
300g cooked beetroot, cut into
    wedges
2 spring onions, trimmed and
    thinly sliced
30g feta cheese
15g nibbed pistachios or
    toasted walnuts (or use
    regular pistachio kernels)
Sea salt and freshly ground
    black pepper

1 Cook the farro in boiling salted water according to the packet instructions for about 10 minutes, until *al dente* (tender but still with a little bite). When the farro is cooked, add the edamame beans to the pan then immediately drain well.

2 Meanwhile, for the dressing, in a large bowl, whisk together the mustard, lemon juice and extra-virgin olive oil. Season well with salt and pepper.

3 Add the kale to the bowl and massage it into the dressing, using your hands to soften it a little. Add the hot farro and edamame and mix well.

4 Stir through the beetroot and spring onions. Season with salt and pepper to taste, and divide between serving plates. Crumble over the feta and sprinkle the nuts over the salad to serve.

 BONUS Combining three different sources of plant proteins – farro, edamame and pistachios – as well as the feta, this hearty salad is a great vegetarian post-workout choice.

Per serving: *541 cals*
21g protein   *55g carbs*
24g fat   *11g fibre*

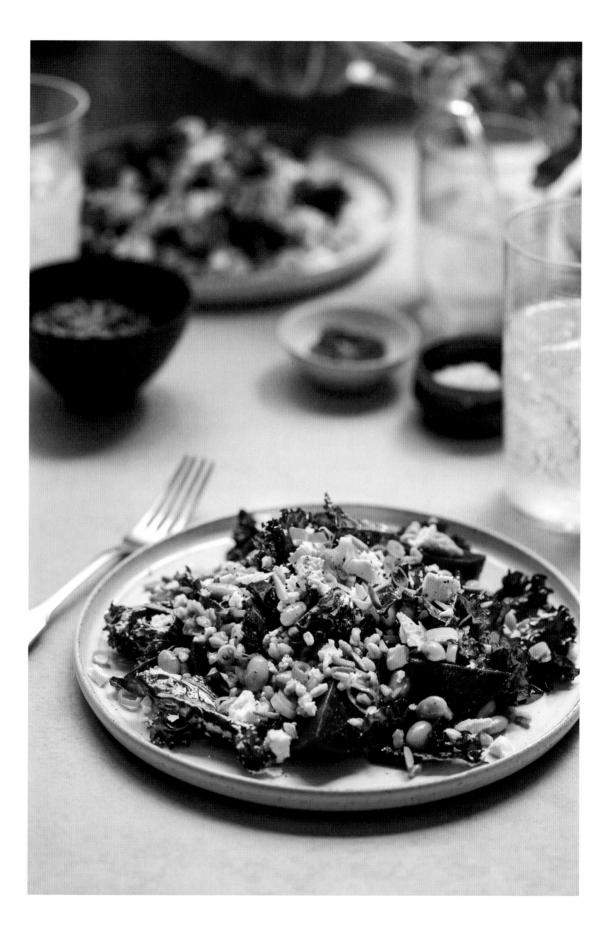

SMOKED MACKEREL PÂTÉ

Make a batch of this creamy smoked mackerel pâté and keep it in the fridge for up to three days to use as an alternative to hummus or taramasalata. It's great as a dip for chopped veg or spread on wholegrain toast.

SERVES 2

200g skinned smoked
    mackerel fillet
1 tbsp reduced-fat cream
    cheese
60ml half-fat crème fraîche
1 tsp creamed horseradish
Finely grated zest of ½ lemon
1 tbsp finely chopped dill
1 tbsp (15g) baby capers
1 tbsp finely chopped basil
Sea salt and freshly ground
    black pepper

For the quick cucumber pickle

½ cucumber, deseeded and
    finely diced
2 tbsp white wine vinegar
½ tsp granulated sweetener
1 tbsp finely chopped dill

For the crudités

4 baby cucumbers (160g),
    halved lengthways
8 baby carrots (140g), scrubbed
12 radishes (120g)
1 Little Gem lettuce, quartered
    lengthways
12 cherry tomatoes, halved

1 First, prepare the quick cucumber pickle: mix all the ingredients together in a bowl along with a little pinch of salt. Cover and refrigerate.

2 To make the pâté, flake the smoked mackerel into a bowl and add all the remaining ingredients. Mix well to combine – you're looking for a rough, slightly flaky texture, not a smooth pâté. Season with a little salt and pepper to taste.

3 Spoon the pâté into 2 serving bowls. Drain the pickled cucumber and spoon on top of the pâté. Place the bowls of pâté on large serving plates and arrange the crudités alongside to serve.

Per serving: *443 cals*
26g protein   *11g carbs*
31g fat   *5g fibre*

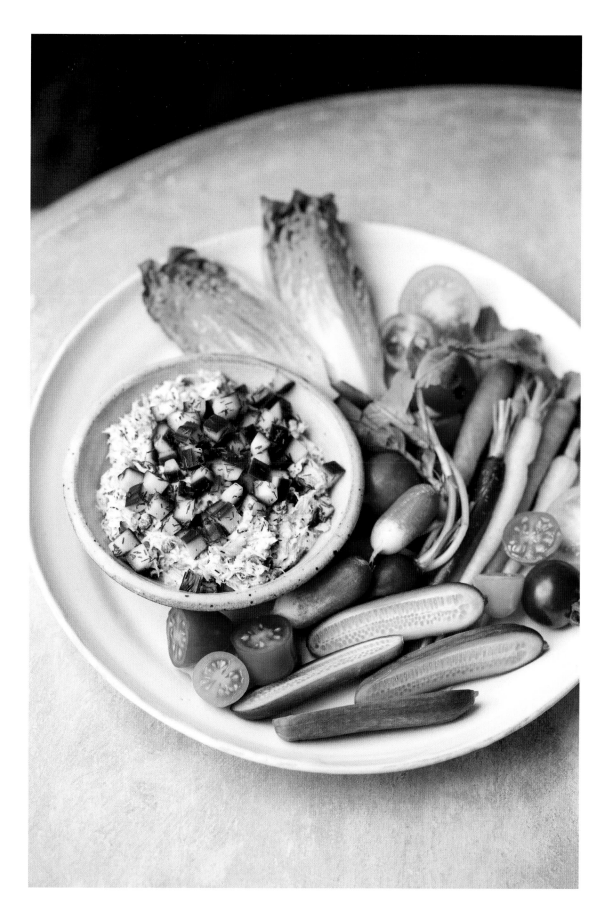

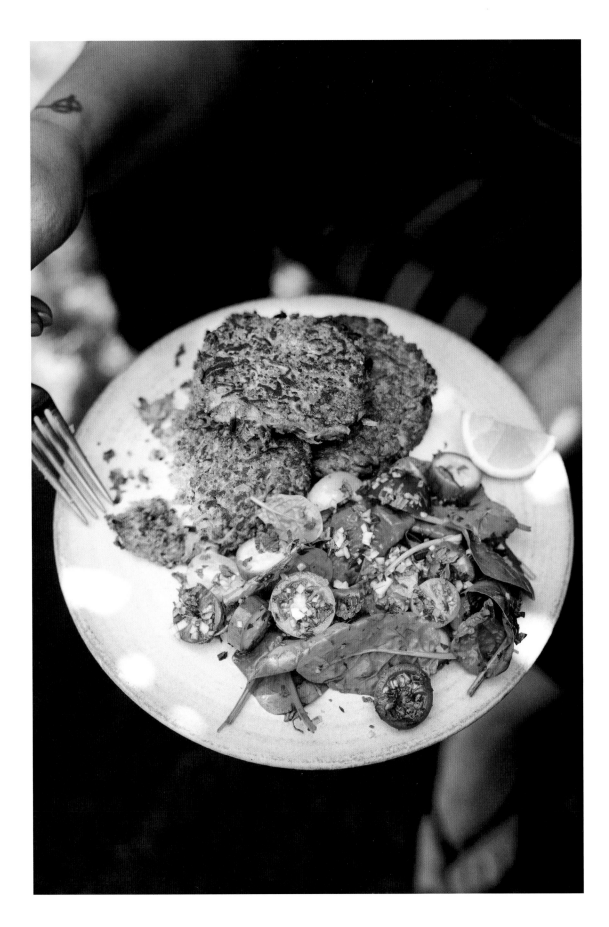

CARROT AND QUINOA FRITTERS

With big, bold North African flavourings from the spices and protein-rich quinoa, these fritters are substantial and filling but don't leave you feeling like you've overeaten – they're a bit like large falafel. All you need is this simple salad on the side. ♡ ❄

SERVES 2

200g carrots, grated
    (prepared weight)
150g sweet potato, grated
    (prepared weight)
2 garlic cloves, grated
1 tsp ground cumin
1 tsp ras el hanout
2 spring onions, finely sliced
2 tbsp chickpea flour
2 large free-range eggs, beaten
250g cooked quinoa (freshly
    cooked and well drained or
    a pouch)
1-cal sunflower oil spray
Sea salt and freshly ground
    black pepper

For the spinach salad

½ red onion, finely chopped
80g spinach leaves
80g cherry tomatoes, halved
2 baby cucumbers, sliced
2 tsp pomegranate molasses
Juice of ½ lemon
A small handful each of mint
    leaves and flat-leaf parsley,
    finely chopped

To serve
Lemon wedges

Per serving: 553 cals
24g protein   77g carbs
13g fat   16g fibre

1 Preheat the oven to 200°C/Fan 180°C/Gas 6. Line a baking tray with a silicone mat or baking paper.

2 Place the grated carrots and sweet potato in a clean tea towel and squeeze out as much liquid as possible. Tip the grated veg into a large bowl. Add the garlic, cumin, ras el hanout, spring onions, chickpea flour, eggs and quinoa. Season well with salt and pepper and mix thoroughly.

3 Divide the mixture into 6 equal pieces and form each into a patty. Heat a large non-stick frying pan over a medium heat, spray the surface with oil and gently place the patties in the pan. Cook for 2 minutes on each side, spraying with more oil as you turn them over. Transfer the patties to the lined tray, spray with more oil and cook in the oven for 10 minutes.

4 In the meantime, prepare the salad. Place all the ingredients in a large bowl, toss to combine and season with salt and pepper to taste.

5 Place 3 fritters on each plate with a portion of salad and a lemon wedge alongside.

TO FREEZE Allow the cooked fritters to cool, then wrap each one separately in foil or cling film. Unwrap and defrost fully in the fridge, then eat the fritters at room temperature or spray with a little more oil and reheat in an oven preheated to 200°C/Fan 180°C/Gas 6 for 5 minutes or until hot through.

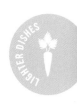

LIGHTER DISHES

CHICKPEA SCOTCH EGGS

Made with a spiced chickpea coating instead of sausage meat, these Scotch eggs have a fantastic flavour. Aim for the egg yolks inside to be a little runny. Delicious eaten while still warm, the eggs are also good cold – pack one into your lunchbox to take to work. ♡

SERVES 6

8 large free-range eggs
2 courgettes, grated
1 tbsp olive oil
1 onion, finely diced
3 garlic cloves, finely chopped
2.5cm piece fresh ginger, grated
2 long green chillies, deseeded and finely chopped
1 tsp ground cumin
1 tsp ground coriander
1 tsp ground turmeric
50g dried onion flakes
50g panko breadcrumbs
2 x 400g tins chickpeas, drained and rinsed
1-cal sunflower oil spray
Sea salt and freshly ground black pepper
Mixed salad leaves, to serve

1 Bring a medium saucepan of water to the boil over a medium-high heat. Carefully lower 6 eggs into the water and cook for 4½ minutes. Lift out the eggs, tap the shells lightly (to make them easier to peel) and immerse in a bowl of cold water to cool.

2 Meanwhile, place the grated courgettes in a clean cloth and squeeze out any excess liquid.

3 Heat the oil in a medium non-stick frying pan over a high heat. When hot, add the onion and cook for 4–5 minutes or until lightly golden. Add the garlic, ginger and chillies and cook for 2 minutes. Sprinkle in the spices and cook, stirring, for 1 minute. Add the grated courgettes to the pan and cook for 2 minutes, stirring from time to time. Remove from the heat and leave to cool slightly.

4 Put the dried onion flakes into a food processor and blitz until they resemble breadcrumbs. Tip them into a shallow bowl, add the panko breadcrumbs and stir to combine.

5 Tip the chickpeas into the food processor and blitz until roughly mashed. Add the courgette and onion mixture and pulse a couple of times to mix. Scrape into a bowl and season generously with salt and pepper to taste.

Per serving: 306 cals
18g protein 27g carbs
13g fat 7g fibre

Continued overleaf

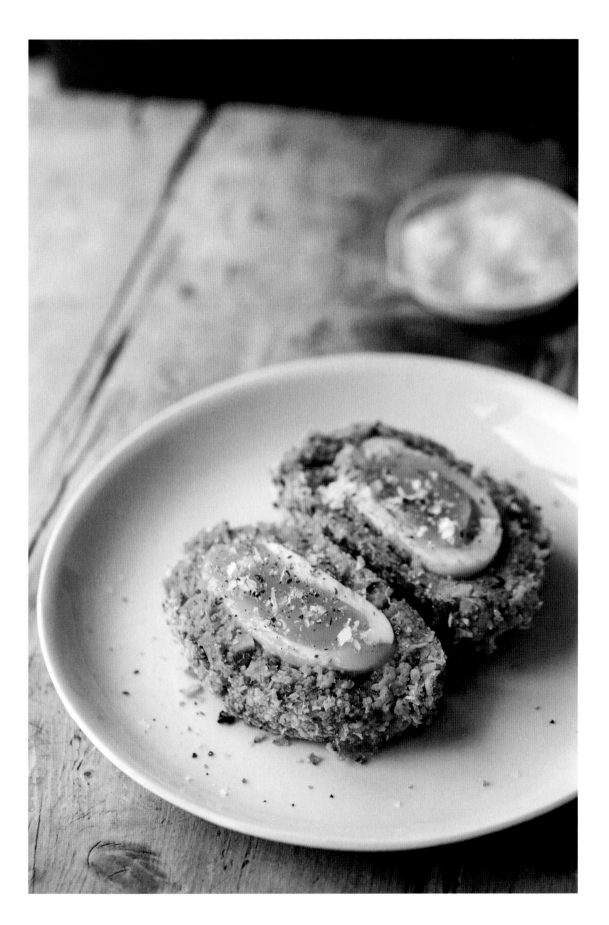

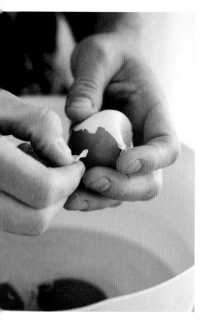

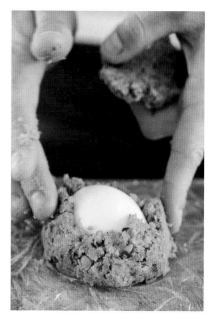

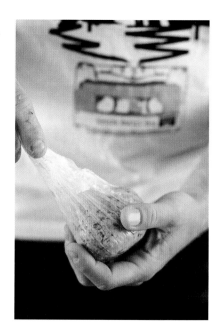

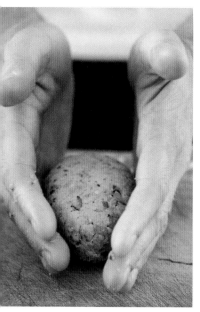

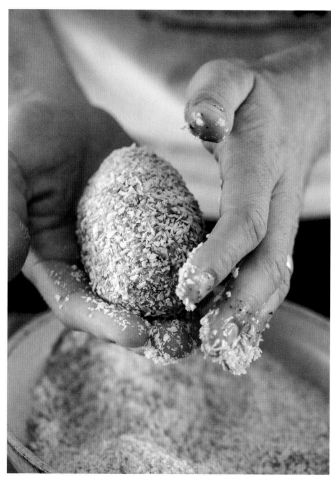

6 Carefully peel the shells from the eggs. Divide the chickpea mixture into 6 equal portions.

7 Lay a piece of cling film (about 20 x 20cm) on a work surface. Place a portion of chickpea mix in the centre and press it out evenly to about a 1cm thickness. Place an egg in the middle and lift the cling film up around it. Gently mould the chickpea mixture around the egg to create an even covering. Repeat with the rest of the shelled eggs and chickpea mixture. Place on a plate and chill in the fridge for at least 1 hour to firm up the coating.

8 Preheat the oven to 220°C/Fan 200°C/Gas 7. Line a baking tray with a silicone mat or baking paper.

9 In a shallow bowl, using a fork, beat the remaining 2 eggs with some salt and pepper. Dip each chickpea egg into the beaten egg and then roll in the crumb mixture to coat all over. Repeat with the other eggs and place on the lined tray.

10 Spray the coated eggs liberally with oil and cook on a high shelf in the oven for 10–12 minutes, then place under a hot grill for a couple of minutes to brown evenly, turning as necessary. Let the chickpea Scotch eggs rest for a few minutes before serving, with a mixed salad on the side.

CHICKEN AND SPINACH BAKED SAMOSAS

These little pastry parcels are packed with flavour and crunch, but they are baked in the oven so they're healthier than regular deep-fried samosas. Minced chicken (or turkey) is much leaner than the usual lamb filling and an easy way to reduce calories.

MAKES 14

2 tsp olive oil
2 onions, finely chopped
3 garlic cloves, finely chopped
5cm piece fresh ginger, finely grated
2 tbsp garam masala
500g chicken (or turkey) thigh mince
250g cooked Puy lentils (freshly cooked and drained or a pouch)
120g baby spinach, roughly chopped
270g packet chilled filo pastry (7 sheets, each 48 x 25cm)
1-cal sunflower oil spray
Sea salt and freshly ground black pepper
Mixed salad leaves, to serve

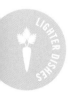

Per samosa: 153 cals
14g protein   14g carbs
4g fat   2g fibre

1 Heat the oil in a large non-stick frying pan over a medium heat. When hot, add the onions and cook for 5 minutes until light golden. Add the garlic and ginger and cook for 2 minutes. Stir in the garam masala and cook, stirring, for 2 minutes.

2 Add the chicken (or turkey) mince, season well with salt and pepper and cook for 5 minutes, breaking it up with a wooden spoon as it cooks.

3 Now add the lentils and spinach and stir well for 2–3 minutes until the spinach is wilted. Season with salt and pepper to taste and leave to cool completely.

4 Preheat the oven to 220°C/Fan 200°C/Gas 7. Line 2 baking trays with silicone mats or baking paper. Cut the filo sheets in half, to give 2 long rectangles (14 strips in total). Keep the filo you aren't working with covered with a lightly dampened clean tea towel.

5 Lay a filo rectangle on your work surface with a short edge facing you and spray it well with oil. Place 3 tbsp of filling at the bottom left-hand corner and shape it into a rough triangle. Fold over the right half of the filo sheet, then fold the bottom left corner over the filo-covered filling to make a triangle. Keep folding over and upwards, forming triangles until you reach the top. Seal with a little oil spray. Repeat with the rest of the filling and pastry. Place on the lined baking trays.

6 Spray the samosas liberally on both sides with oil. Cook in the oven for 10–15 minutes or until evenly golden brown. Serve with the salad leaves.

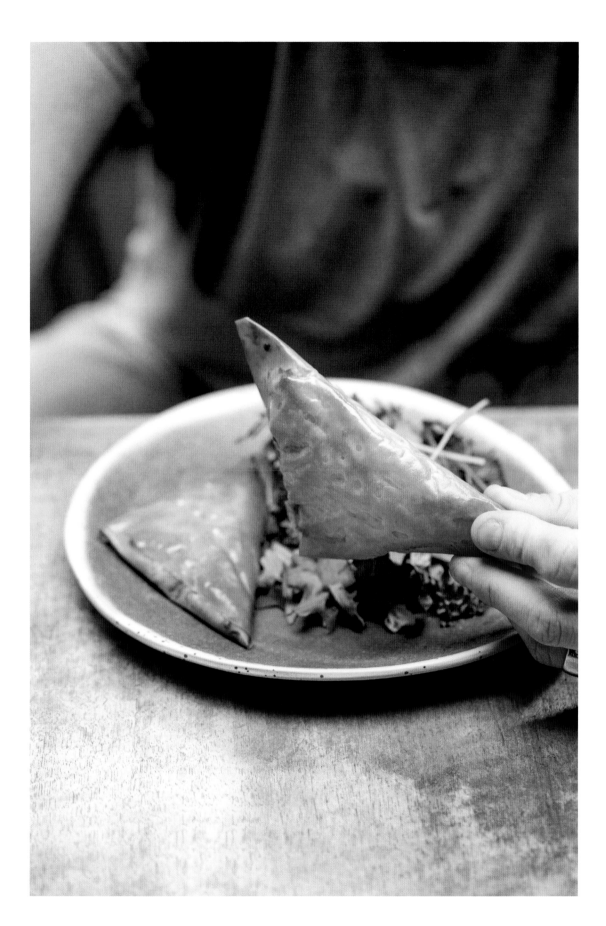

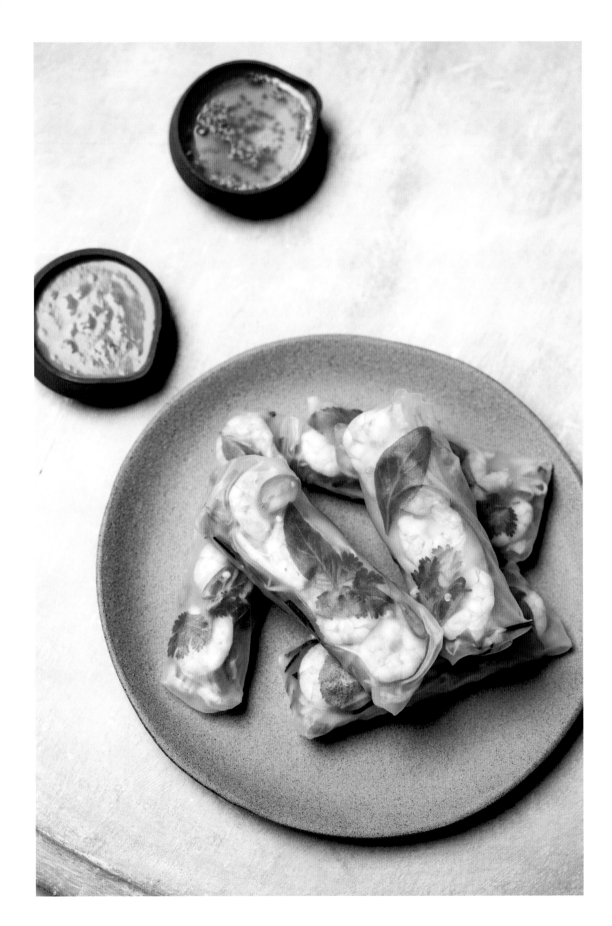

PRAWN AND AVOCADO RICE PAPER ROLLS

Packed with flavour and texture, these rice paper wraps are great as a packed lunch. The dipping sauces – a sweet and sour nuoc cham and a tasty peanut sauce – make them extra special. Try using strips of cooked chicken breast instead of the prawns.

MAKES 8

8 large rice paper spring roll wrappers (22cm diameter)
1 long red chilli, finely sliced
A small handful each of Thai basil, coriander and mint leaves
200g cooked peeled prawns
100g cucumber, julienned
100g carrot, julienned
100g beansprouts
100g Iceberg lettuce, shredded
80g red cabbage, finely shredded
1 ripe avocado, thinly sliced

For the nuoc cham
½ red chilli, finely diced
20ml fish sauce
20ml rice vinegar
1 tsp granulated sweetener
2 tbsp water
Juice of ½ lime
1 garlic clove, finely chopped

For the peanut dipping sauce
1 tbsp peanut butter
1 tsp hoisin sauce
1 tsp sesame oil
2 tbsp rice vinegar
1–2 tsp water

Per roll: *125 cals*
6g protein   *11g carbs*
6g fat   *2g fibre*

1 Have all your ingredients prepared and laid out in front of you, ready to roll.

2 Fill a shallow bowl or lipped plate with warm water, big enough to dip the rice paper wrappers into. Gently dip a rice paper into the water for a few seconds and then lay it on a work surface.

3 Place a couple of slices of red chilli on the third of the rice paper closest to you. Top with a few fresh herbs and 3 or 4 prawns. Cover with some cucumber and carrot julienne, beansprouts, shredded lettuce and cabbage, and 1 or 2 avocado slices.

4 Start rolling the rice paper over the filling, tucking in the two sides and rolling the wrapper tightly around the filling. Repeat with the rest of the wrappers and filling ingredients.

5 For the nuoc cham, mix all the ingredients together in a small bowl. For the peanut dipping sauce, mix the ingredients together in another bowl, adding 1–2 tsp water to loosen the mix to the desired consistency.

6 Serve the rice paper rolls with the nuoc cham and peanut dipping sauces.

CHARGRILLED SARDINES WITH BEETROOT SLAW

The rich, oily taste of sardines is amazing alongside this earthy slaw. When they are in season, sardines are incredible – simply cook them whole and then peel off the flesh from the bones. They are pretty hard to overcook because of their healthy fat content so they're great if you happen to be nervous about cooking with fish.

SERVES 2

6 sardines (60g each), gutted
1-cal olive oil spray
Sea salt and freshly ground
    black pepper

For the beetroot slaw
1 beetroot, grated
    (60g prepared weight)
1 carrot, grated
    (90g prepared weight)
½ small fennel, finely shredded
    (50g prepared weight)
A small wedge of red cabbage,
    finely shredded
    (80g prepared weight)
1 tbsp light mayonnaise
1 tbsp reduced-fat soured
    cream
1 tbsp apple cider vinegar
1 tsp Dijon mustard
1 tbsp roughly chopped dill,
    plus a few extra fronds
    to finish

To serve
Lemon wedges

1 First, prepare the slaw. Put the beetroot, carrot, fennel and cabbage into a medium bowl. In a small bowl, mix together the mayonnaise, soured cream, cider vinegar, mustard and dill. Add the dressing to the vegetables and toss to coat them well, seasoning with salt and pepper to taste.

2 Place a non-stick griddle over a medium-high heat. Season both sides of the sardines with salt and pepper and spray them all over with oil.

3 Once the griddle is hot, lay the sardines on it and cook for 2–4 minutes on each side, until charred on the outside and cooked through.

4 Divide the slaw between serving plates and place the sardines on top. Add a lemon wedge to each plate and serve at once.

 BONUS Sardines are an excellent source of healthy omega-3 fatty acids, which have powerful anti-inflammatory properties and help your body to recover after exercise.

Per serving: *322 cals*
38g protein   *8g carbs*
14g fat   *5g fibre*

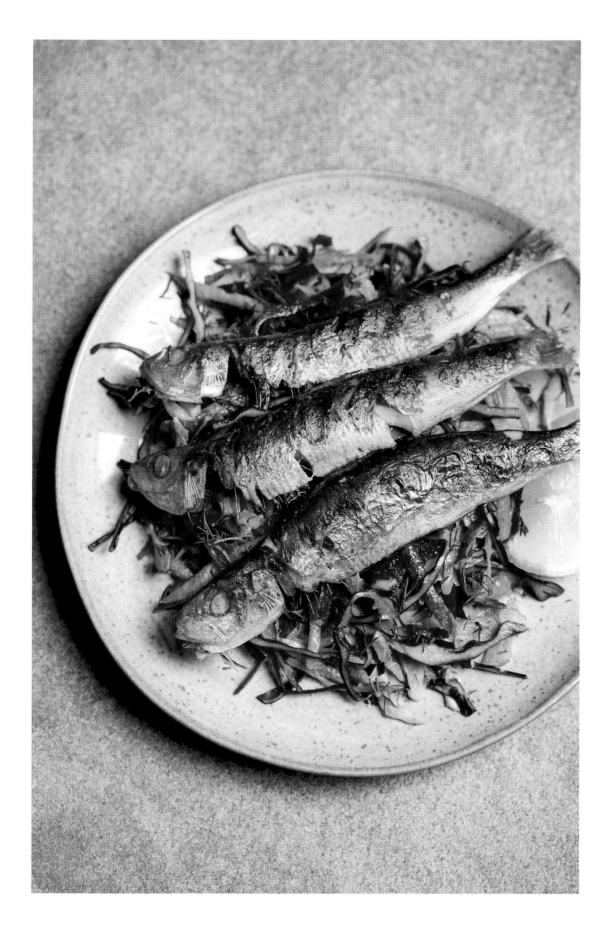

CAULIFLOWER QUINOA COUSCOUS

Cauliflower helps to bulk out this fresh-tasting quinoa salad and up the fibre content without adding loads of extra calories. It makes a delicious, quick, light dinner, or you could serve it as a healthy side dish for a curry. ♡

SERVES 2

250g cauliflower
1 tsp olive oil
1 red onion (90g), diced
400g tin chickpeas, drained and rinsed (240g drained weight)
1 tsp hot Madras curry powder
½ tsp ground turmeric
¼ tsp ground cinnamon
150ml fresh vegetable stock
250g cooked quinoa (freshly cooked and drained or a pouch)
100g frozen peas
2 baby cucumbers, thickly sliced
A large handful of coriander, roughly chopped
1 lime, halved, to serve

1 Break the cauliflower into florets and pulse in a food processor until it starts to resemble couscous grains.

2 Heat the oil in a large non-stick frying pan over a medium heat. When it is hot, add the onion and chickpeas and cook for about 5 minutes until the onion is starting to brown. If the pan appears to be drying out, add a splash of water.

3 Sprinkle in the spices and cook for 1 minute, then pour in the stock and add the cauliflower 'couscous'. Cook until the stock has evaporated completely. Remove from the heat.

4 Tip the cooked quinoa into the pan, along with the frozen peas and stir well until the peas have defrosted. Season generously with salt and pepper.

5 Stir through the sliced cucumbers and half the coriander. Spoon the quinoa couscous into warmed bowls and sprinkle with the remaining coriander. Serve with the lime halves for squeezing.

Per serving: *530 cals*
24g protein   *71g carbs*
12g fat   *19g fibre*

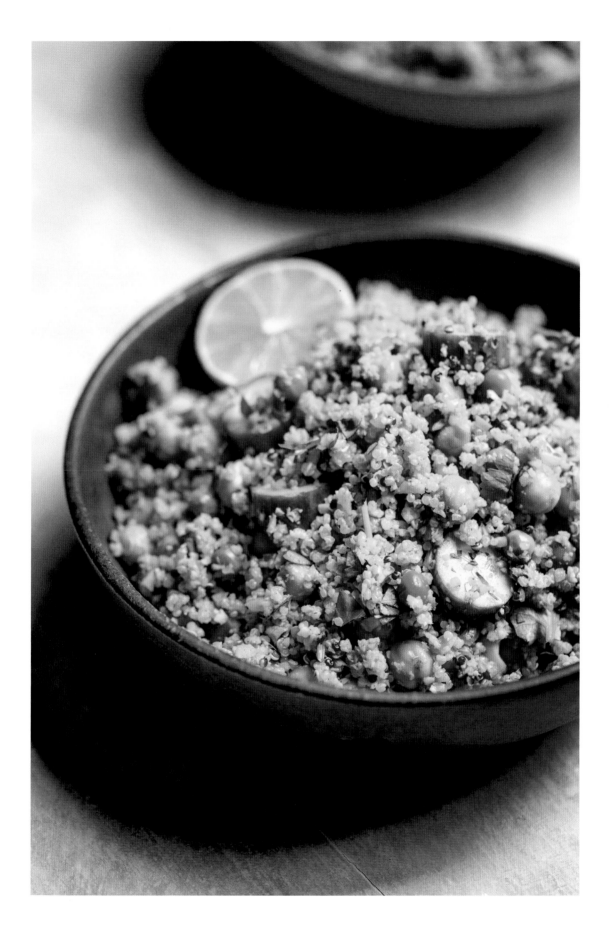

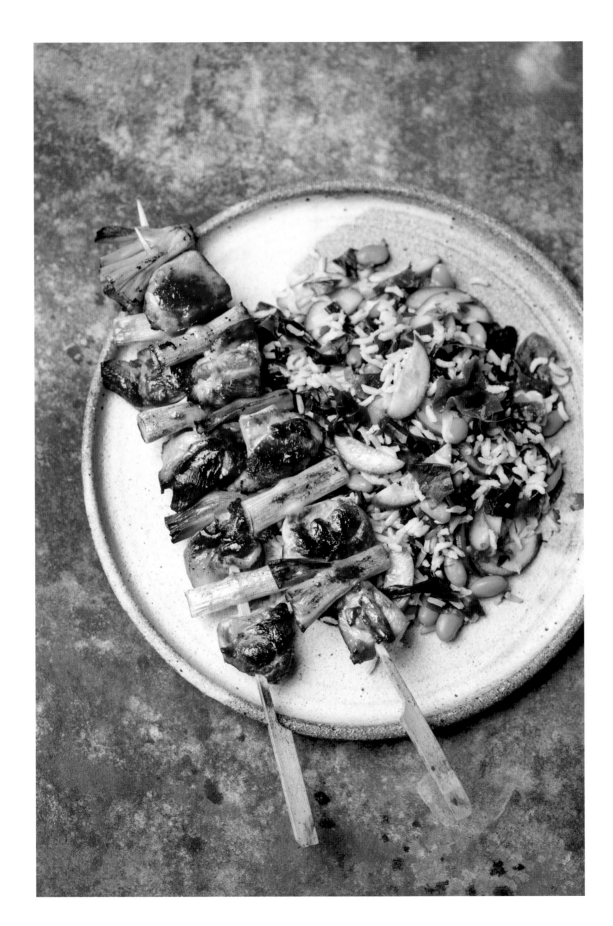

CHICKEN YAKITORI

I ate something similar to this at a restaurant called Yard Bird in Hong Kong, which specialises in yakitori skewers that use every single bit of the chicken – including the knee caps. My version uses chicken thighs only and it's served with a seaweed rice salad. Seaweed has a lovely salty, umami flavour – give it a go!

SERVES 2

4 skinless boneless chicken thighs
6 spring onions, cut into 4cm lengths

For the marinade
2 tbsp soy sauce
2 tbsp mirin
1 tbsp sake
1 tsp light brown sugar

For the brown rice salad
10g (about 2 tbsp) wakame
250g cooked brown rice (freshly cooked and drained or a pouch)
2 baby cucumbers, halved lengthways
100g frozen edamame beans, defrosted
2 tbsp pickled ginger, shredded
A small handful of coriander, roughly chopped
1 tsp soy sauce
1 tsp sesame oil
2 tsp white miso
Juice of ½ lime
1-cal sunflower oil spray

Per serving: 632 cals
45g protein   53g carbs
26g fat   5g fibre

1 Pre-soak 4 wooden skewers in a tray of water.

2 For the marinade, mix the ingredients together in a medium bowl. Cut each chicken thigh into 6 even-sized pieces. Add to the marinade and mix well. Set aside in the fridge until needed.

3 To prepare the rice salad, put the wakame into a small heatproof bowl, cover with boiling water and set aside to rehydrate for 5–10 minutes.

4 Tip the cooked rice into a large bowl (heating it up first according to the packet instructions if necessary). Cut the cucumbers into thin half-moons and add to the bowl along with the edamame beans, pickled ginger, coriander, soy sauce, sesame oil, miso and lime juice. Drain the wakame and if it isn't already chopped, cut into bite-sized pieces before adding to the salad. Mix well.

5 Thread the marinated chicken onto the skewers, alternating each chunk with a piece of spring onion.

6 Place a non-stick griddle pan on a high heat. Spray the skewers a few times all over with oil. Once the griddle is smoking hot, add the skewers and cook for 3–4 minutes on each side, then brush each skewer with the marinade and cook for a further 2 minutes on each side or until the chicken is cooked through.

7 Divide the rice salad between plates and place the chicken skewers alongside to serve.

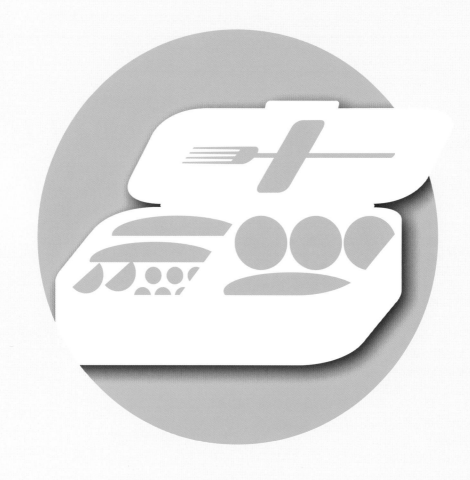

3 MEAL PREP

TO MAKE HEALTHY EATING sustainable in the long term, you need to make life as easy as possible for yourself. Be prepared for those moments of weakness, so you won't be tempted to give in to cravings or use those old excuses of being too tired, too busy or not having the right ingredients in your cupboards. When you start to make better choices for yourself, it's important to arm yourself with as much information as you can – knowledge is key.

I've learned that a healthy plate of food should include unrefined carbs to provide a steady amount of energy throughout the day and to replace the sugars that you use up during exercise. These include brown rice, quinoa, sweet potato and wholewheat pasta. There should also be a good amount of lean protein, such as chicken, turkey, fish, prawns, eggs, lean red meat, tofu, lentils or chickpeas, to keep you feeling full and to help your body recover. Alongside these should be a generous serving of colourful fruit or veg, and some healthy fats (a few nuts or seeds, avocado or olive oil, perhaps).

The recipes in this chapter are all perfectly balanced so they support your weight loss and improved fitness. The idea is that you can make the recipe, portion it into containers in the fridge and then eat it over the next couple of days. It means you won't need to cook on your busier days and you'll be less likely to make unhealthy choices because you're hungry and in a rush. Try the delicious sticky teriyaki salmon on page 90 or my peri peri chicken on page 96. Make some for dinner and then enjoy the rest for lunch the next day. Most of the recipes are fine to eat cold, but you may prefer to reheat them for lunch if you have the facility to do so. If you'll be using a microwave for reheating, remember to pack the meal in a suitable, non-metal container.

I think well-balanced meals need to be equally well-balanced in terms of taste too. I'm always looking for easy ways to add extra layers of flavour and texture without driving up the calorie count. I like to make use of powerfully flavoured ingredients, such as citrus fruits, gherkins and pickles, which are quick ways to add a little acidity to lift a recipe. The quick pickled red onions in the burrito bowls on page 92 add a much-needed sharpness as well as an amazing pink colour. And the spice rub on the Cajun salmon on page 99 is another instant way to boost flavour without racking up calories.

The recipes in this chapter offer delicious, healthy alternatives to shop-bought ready meals. Use these as the basis to start experimenting with your own meal prep boxes. You might be short on time, but that doesn't mean you need to compromise on taste and satisfaction.

KOREAN-STYLE GRILLED LAMB

Korean cooking is high in flavour and the marinade for this lamb has some bold spicing going on! Lamb is robust in terms of both taste and texture, so it can stand up to strong flavours. Grilling meat like this is an easy way to cut back on calories.

SERVES 4

4 lean lamb leg steaks, trimmed of any fat (150g each), at room temperature

For the marinade
3 tbsp gochujang (red chilli paste)
1 tbsp soy sauce
1 tbsp mirin
2 garlic cloves, grated
2.5cm piece fresh ginger, finely grated

For the sesame green beans
400g green beans, cut in half
2 tbsp tahini
1½ tbsp rice vinegar
1 tsp sesame oil
A pinch of granulated sweetener
1 tbsp water
Sea salt and freshly ground black pepper

To serve
500g cooked wholegrain rice and quinoa (freshly cooked and drained or 2 pouches)
2 spring onions, julienned
1 tsp black sesame seeds

Per serving: *605 cals*
38g protein   *46g carbs*
28g fat   *9g fibre*

1. Preheat the oven to 240°C/Fan 220°C/Gas 9 with the grill element on.

2. In a medium bowl, mix together the ingredients for the marinade. Add the lamb steaks and turn to coat well on both sides. Leave to marinate for 2 hours if you have time, or at least while you cook the beans.

3. Bring a medium saucepan of salted water to the boil. Add the green beans and cook for 3–4 minutes or until tender. Drain the beans in a colander and run them under cold water to stop the cooking process.

4. Lay the lamb steaks on a baking tray and grill on a high shelf in the oven for 4–5 minutes on each side. Take out of the oven and run a cook's blowtorch over both sides to char lightly. Leave to rest for 2–3 minutes.

5. Meanwhile, if using pouches of rice and quinoa and serving straight away, heat up according to the packet instructions.

6. In a bowl, mix together the tahini, rice vinegar, sesame oil, sweetener and water. Add the beans and stir to coat. Season with salt and pepper to taste.

7. Divide the rice and quinoa between 4 bowls or containers. Slice the lamb and arrange on top. Add the beans and sprinkle with the spring onions and sesame seeds. Serve at once, or cool then seal the container and keep in the fridge. Eat within 2 days, either cold or reheated (lift off and set aside the spring onions before reheating).

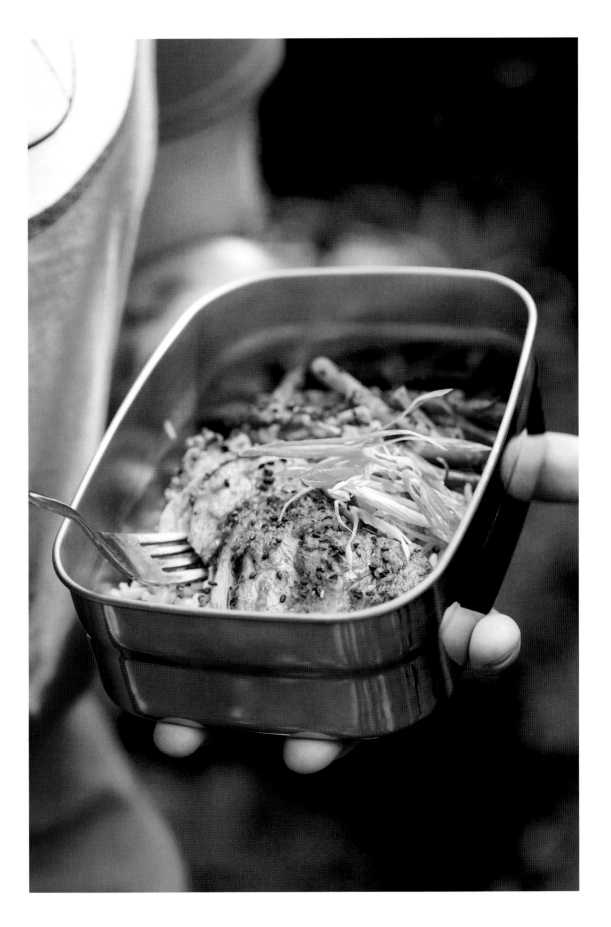

TERIYAKI SALMON

Frying this salmon in its marinade creates a sweet, sticky glaze. It's definitely not what you'd expect to be eating when you are on a diet! The pickled radishes provide the perfect counterbalance to the richness of the fish.

SERVES 4

200g broccoli, cut into small florets
150g frozen edamame beans
4 salmon fillets (180g each), skin on

For the teriyaki sauce

3 tbsp soy sauce
2 garlic cloves, finely grated
2cm piece fresh ginger, finely grated
3 tbsp mirin
75ml apple juice

For the pickled radishes

8 radishes, cut into quarters
2 tbsp rice vinegar
A pinch of granulated sweetener

To serve

500g cooked brown rice (freshly cooked and drained or 2 pouches)
4 spring onions, green part only, finely shredded
1 tsp toasted sesame seeds

Per serving: 653 cals
53g protein   52g carbs
25g fat   6g fibre

1. First mix all the ingredients for the teriyaki sauce together in a small bowl and set aside.

2. Put the radishes, rice vinegar and sweetener into another bowl. Mix well and leave for 10 minutes to pickle slightly.

3. Place the broccoli florets in a steamer over boiling water and steam for 4–5 minutes. Add the edamame beans and steam for a further 1–2 minutes, then remove from the steamer.

4. While the broccoli is cooking, pat the salmon dry with kitchen paper. Place a large non-stick frying pan over a medium-high heat. When hot, add the salmon fillets, skin side down, and cook for 3 minutes. Flip the salmon over in the pan, add the teriyaki sauce and cook for a further 2 minutes, or until the sauce has reduced to a glaze and the salmon is cooked. (If your pan isn't big enough to take all 4 fillets, cook them two at a time.)

5. Meanwhile, if using pouches of rice and serving right away, heat up according to the packet instructions.

6. Divide the rice between 4 bowls or containers. Top with the salmon, broccoli and edamame, pickled radishes and spring onions. Finally, sprinkle with the toasted sesame seeds. Serve at once, or cool then seal and keep in the fridge. Eat within 2 days, either cold or reheated (lift off and set aside the pickled radishes and spring onions before reheating).

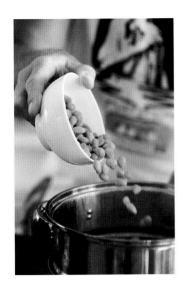
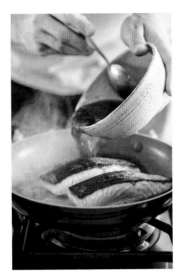
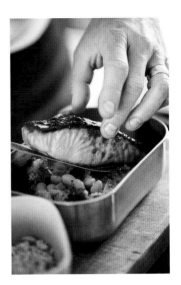
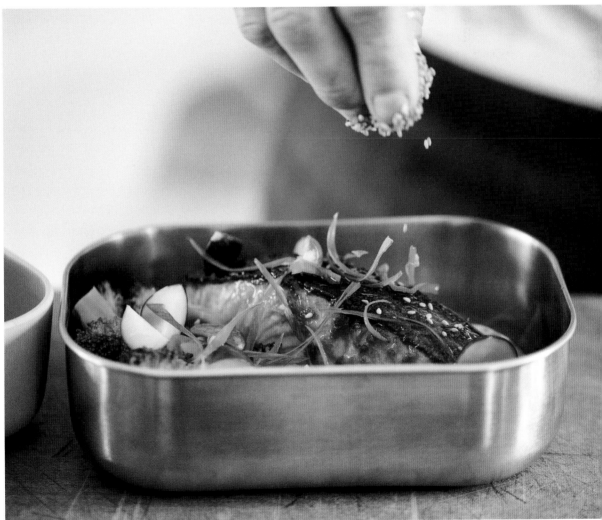

CORN AND BLACK BEAN BURRITO BOWLS

There is so much going on in these veg-based bowls. Black beans and sweetcorn are peppered with jalapeños and cumin, while red onions quickly pickled in lime juice provide a refreshing, sharp finish. For less heat, leave out the pickled jalapeños. ♡

SERVES 4

2 tsp olive oil
2 red onions, diced
4 garlic cloves, finely chopped
2 fresh jalapeño peppers, finely
    chopped (with seeds)
1 tsp hot smoked paprika
2 tsp ground cumin
3 tbsp tomato purée
600ml fresh vegetable stock
2 x 400g tins black beans
325g tin sweetcorn, drained
    (260g drained weight)
1 tsp dried oregano
2 green peppers, cored,
    deseeded and diced
A large handful of coriander,
    finely chopped
80g pickled jalapeño peppers
Sea salt and freshly ground
    black pepper

For the pickled red onion

1 red onion
Juice of 2 limes
½ tsp dried oregano

To serve

500g cooked brown and wild
    rice (freshly cooked and
    drained or 2 pouches)

Per serving: *516 cals*
20g protein   *83g carbs*
8g fat   *17g fibre*

1 Heat the oil in a large non-stick saucepan over a high heat. Add the onions and cook for 3–4 minutes to soften, then add the garlic and jalapeños and cook for 2 minutes. Stir in the spices, cook for 1 minute, then add the tomato purée and cook, stirring, for 2 minutes.

2 Meanwhile, for the pickled onion, halve and thinly slice the onion. Put into a heatproof bowl, cover with boiling water and leave to stand for 10 minutes.

3 Pour the stock into the saucepan, stir well and bring to a simmer. Drain and rinse the beans under cold running water, then add to the pan with the drained sweetcorn and dried oregano. Season well with salt and pepper and simmer gently for 10 minutes.

4 In the meantime, drain the soaked red onion in a sieve and return it to the bowl. Add the lime juice along with the dried oregano and a good pinch of salt. Mix well and leave for another 10 minutes.

5 Add the green peppers to the beans, stir well and cook for another 5 minutes. Now stir through the coriander.

6 Meanwhile, if using pouches of rice and serving right away, heat up according to the packet instructions.

7 Divide the rice between 4 bowls or containers. Spoon the beans and corn next to the rice. Top with the pickled onion and jalapeños. Serve at once, or cool then seal and keep in the fridge. Eat within 2 days, either cold or reheated (lift off and set aside the pickled onions and jalapeños before reheating).

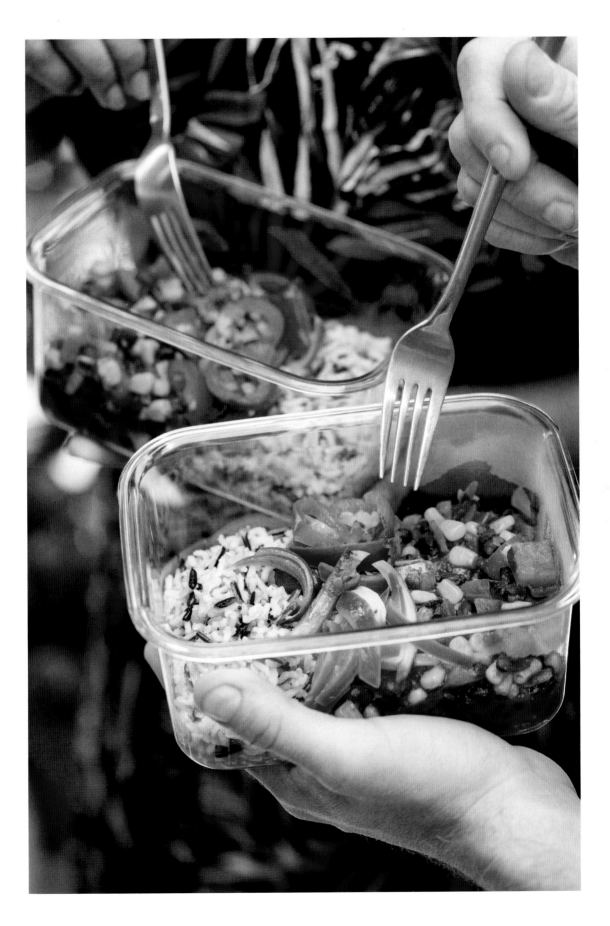

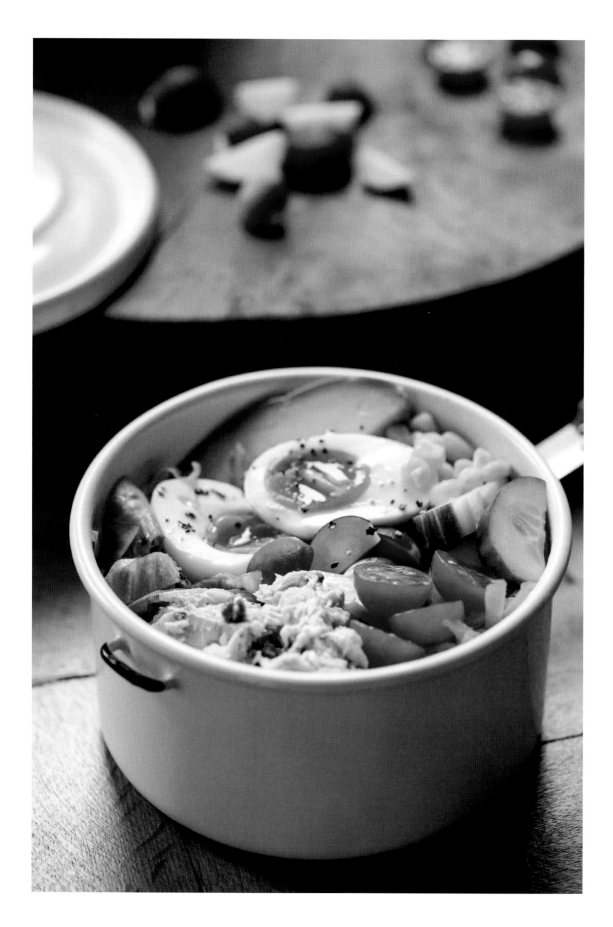

TUNA COBB SALAD BOWL

This is a good example of the kind of salad that you can throw together using ingredients that might already be in the cupboard and fridge. Feel free to swap things around depending on what you have. The one thing I'd say you need to keep is the baby capers – they may be tiny but they add so much flavour.

SERVES 4

4 large free-range eggs
400g tinned tuna in spring water (drained weight)
Juice of ½ lemon, plus an extra squeeze for the avocado
1 tbsp baby capers, rinse
50ml light mayonnaise
350g Iceberg lettuce, shredded
150g carrots, grated
8 cherry tomatoes, halved
½ cucumber, halved lengthways and thickly sliced
200g drained tinned sweetcorn
8 radishes, quartered
1 ripe avocado, peeled, quartered and stoned
Sea salt and freshly ground black pepper

For the dressing
3 tbsp extra-virgin olive oil
1½ tbsp red wine vinegar
1 tsp Dijon mustard

1 Place a small saucepan of water over a high heat and bring to the boil. Carefully add the eggs and cook for 7 minutes. Remove the eggs and immerse them in a bowl of cold water to cool quickly.

2 Flake the tuna and place in a bowl with the lemon juice, capers and mayonnaise. Season with salt and pepper to taste and mix well.

3 Lay out 4 containers and cover the base of each one with shredded lettuce and grated carrot. Top with the tuna mayo, cherry tomatoes, cucumber, sweetcorn and radishes. Squeeze some lemon juice over the avocado slices and add these to the containers.

4 For the dressing, whisk the ingredients together in a small bowl and season with salt and pepper to taste. Spoon over the salads.

5 Peel the cooled boiled eggs, then halve and season with a little salt and pepper. Add the eggs to your containers. Serve straight away or seal and keep in the fridge. Eat within 2 days.

 BONUS The colourful veggies in this salad provide a huge range of nutrients that are anti-inflammatory and help muscles to recover after exercise.

Per serving: *460 cals*
37g protein   *14g carbs*
27g fat   *7g fibre*

PERI PERI CHICKEN

This tasty chicken and spicy rice dish is inspired by my favourite date-night – going to the local peri peri chicken shop and then to the cinema. The slaw is a great versatile side for other dishes too.

SERVES 4

8 skinless boneless chicken
    thighs
75ml medium-hot peri peri
    sauce
½ tsp hot smoked paprika
Sea salt and freshly ground
    black pepper

For the dirty rice

1 red pepper
1 green pepper
1 tsp olive oil
1 red onion, finely chopped
2 garlic cloves, finely chopped
1 tsp paprika
1 tsp ground cumin
A large pinch of saffron strands
200ml fresh chicken stock
1 chicken stock cube
500g cooked brown rice
    (freshly cooked and drained
    or 2 pouches)

For the coleslaw

250g red and/or white
    cabbage, finely shredded
1 carrot, grated (100g
    prepared weight)
2 tbsp Greek yoghurt (0% fat)
2 tbsp white wine vinegar
3 tbsp light mayonnaise

Per serving: *614 cals*
41g protein   *50g carbs*
26g fat   *7g fibre*

1 Preheat the oven to 240°C/Fan 220°C/Gas 9. Line a baking tray with a silicone mat or baking paper.

2 Slash the chicken thighs lightly with a sharp knife and place in a bowl. Add 50ml of the peri peri sauce, the smoked paprika and a little salt and pepper. Turn the chicken to coat well then lay on the lined tray. Cook on the highest shelf of the oven for 20–25 minutes.

3 Meanwhile, prepare the dirty rice. Halve, core, deseed and finely chop the peppers. Place a sauté pan over a high heat and add the oil. When hot, add the onion and cook for 4–5 minutes until starting to brown. Add the peppers and garlic and cook for 2 minutes.

4 Add the paprika and cumin and cook for 1 minute, Grind the saffron with a pestle and mortar and add to the pan with the stock and crumbled stock cube. Simmer for 2–3 minutes, stirring to dissolve the stock cube. Add the rice and warm through for 5 minutes.

5 Meanwhile, mix all the ingredients for the coleslaw together and season with salt and pepper to taste.

6 Remove the chicken from the oven, tip the juices from the tray into the rice and stir through. Cook the rice for a further 2 minutes. Wave a cook's blowtorch over the surface of the chicken thighs to lightly char them, then brush with the remaining peri peri sauce to glaze.

7 Serve the chicken straight away, with the rice and coleslaw. Or cool, pack into containers, seal and keep in the fridge. Eat within 2 days, either cold or reheated (lift off and set aside the coleslaw before reheating).

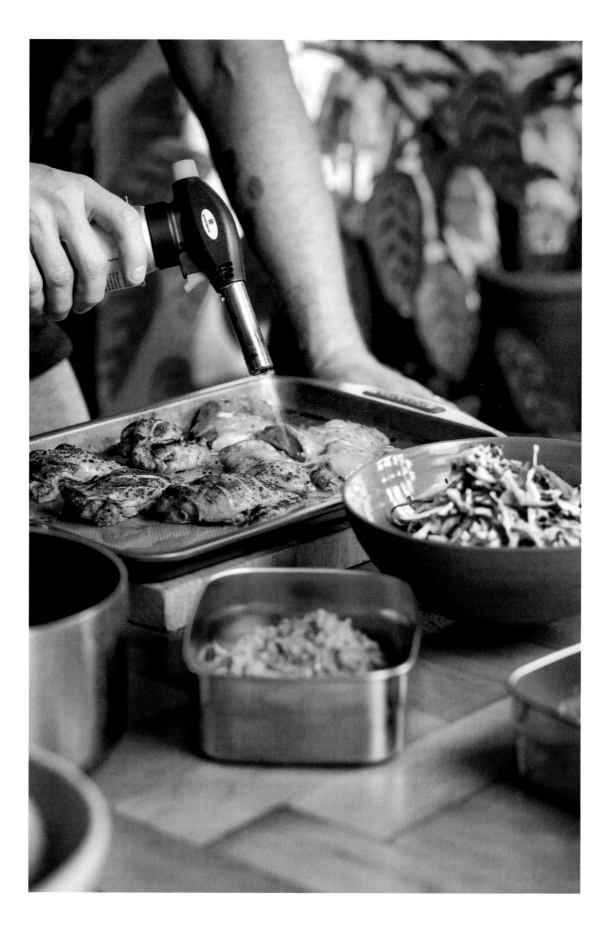

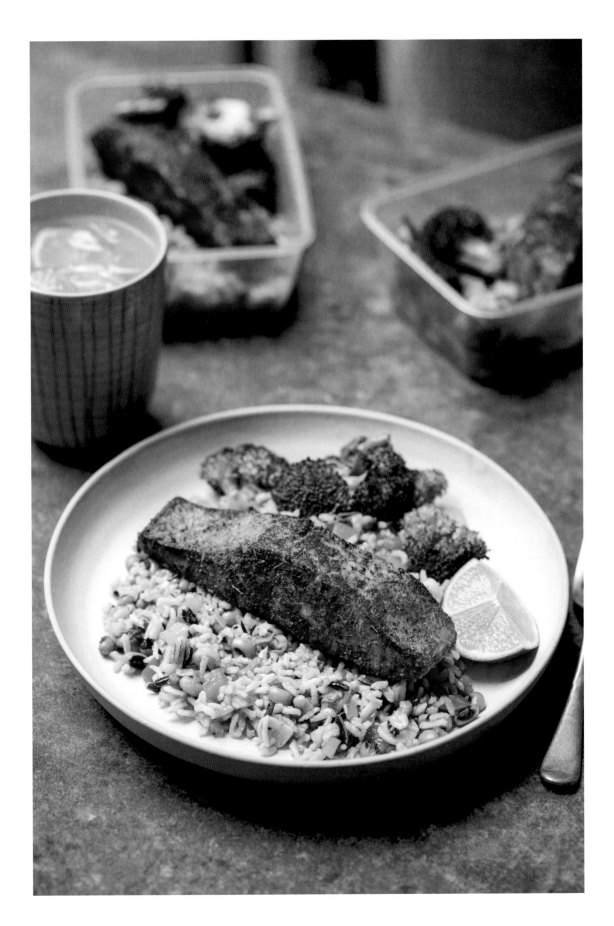

CAJUN SALMON

 POST

Using punchy flavours like Cajun seasoning helps to keep your cooking exciting, taking lower-calorie mealtimes to the next level.

SERVES 4

4 skinless salmon fillets (120g each)
250g (1 small head) broccoli
1-cal sunflower oil spray
Sea salt and freshly ground black pepper

For the Cajun seasoning
1 heaped tsp ground cumin
1 tsp garlic granules
½ tsp hot smoked paprika
½ tsp cayenne pepper
½ tsp dried oregano
½ tsp dried thyme

For the dirty rice
1 tsp olive oil
1 onion, finely diced
2 garlic cloves, sliced
1 red pepper, cored, deseeded and finely diced
1 tbsp tomato purée
1 tsp dried oregano
½ tsp dried thyme
200ml fresh chicken stock
400g tin black eye beans
500g cooked brown and wild rice (freshly cooked and drained or 2 pouches)
4 spring onions, finely sliced

To serve
1 lime, cut into wedges

Per serving: *552 cals*
41g protein   *55g carbs*
17g fat   *9g fibre*

1 Preheat the oven to 200°C/Fan 180°C/Gas 6.

2 For the Cajun seasoning, mix the ingredients together in a small bowl with 1 tsp flaky sea salt. Pat each salmon fillet dry with kitchen paper and then sprinkle with the seasoning on all sides. Leave to marinate while you prepare the broccoli and dirty rice.

3 Line a baking tray with a silicone mat (or spray with oil). Cut the broccoli into bite-sized florets, season with salt and pepper and spread out on the tray. Cook on a high shelf in the oven for 12 minutes or until the broccoli is lightly charred and cooked through.

4 Meanwhile, for the dirty rice, heat the oil in a large sauté pan over a medium heat. When hot, add the onion and cook for 4–5 minutes until softened. Add the garlic and cook for 2 minutes, then add the red pepper and tomato purée and stir well. Add the oregano, thyme and stock and bring to a simmer.

5 Drain the black eye beans and add to the pan with the rice. Cook for another 5 minutes. Season well with salt and pepper and stir through the spring onions.

6 Heat a medium non-stick frying pan over a medium heat. Spray the salmon fillets a few times with oil then place in the pan. Cook for 2–3 minutes on each side or until lightly charred and cooked through.

7 Spoon the rice into 4 shallow bowls or containers and add the broccoli and salmon. Serve at once, with lime wedges. Or cool then seal and keep in the fridge. Eat within 2 days, either cold or reheated.

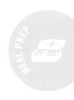

CAULIFLOWER CURRY WITH ROASTED SQUASH

We're all becoming much more aware of veg being more than just a side dish. And if the focus of the dish is as tasty, spicy and flavoursome as this, then long live the cauliflower! ♡ ❄

SERVES 4

400g peeled, deseeded butternut squash, cut into 2cm pieces
1-cal sunflower oil spray
1 tsp vegetable oil
1 tsp black mustard seeds
1 onion, finely diced
2 garlic cloves, finely chopped
2 green chillies, finely chopped (with seeds)
1 tsp ground turmeric
1 tsp ground cumin
1 tsp ground coriander
1 tsp garam masala
500ml fresh vegetable stock
300g cauliflower, cut into small florets
100g green beans, trimmed
2 x 400g tins chickpeas, drained and rinsed (480g total drained weight)
100ml tinned coconut milk
Sea salt and freshly ground black pepper

To serve

500g cooked wholegrain rice (freshly cooked and drained or 2 pouches)

Per serving: 517 cals
19g protein   74g carbs
13g fat   14g fibre

1 Preheat the oven to 240°C/Fan 220°C/Gas 9. Line a baking tray with a silicone mat or baking paper.

2 Spread the butternut squash out on the tray and spray a few times with oil. Season well with salt and pepper. Roast on a high shelf in the oven for 20 minutes or until roasted, tender and golden.

3 Heat the 1 tsp oil in a large sauté pan over a medium-high heat. When hot, toss in the mustard seeds and fry until they begin to pop, then add the onion and cook for 4–5 minutes until it starts to brown. Add the garlic and chillies and cook for 2 minutes. Stir in all the ground spices along with a big pinch of salt and stir well for 1 minute or until they release their aroma.

4 Pour in the stock, bring to a simmer and add the cauliflower. Cook for 4 minutes, then toss in the beans and cook for a further 3–4 minutes. Add the chickpeas and coconut milk and bring back to a simmer to heat through. Season with salt and pepper to taste.

5 Meanwhile, if using pouches of rice and serving right away, heat up according to the packet instructions.

6 Divide the rice between 4 bowls or containers. Spoon the cauliflower curry next to the rice and add the roasted squash. Serve at once, or cool then seal the container and keep in the fridge. Eat within 2 days, either cold or reheated.

TO FREEZE Cool then pack into one- or two-portion tubs and freeze. Defrost fully in the fridge, then reheat in a saucepan over a medium heat or in the microwave.

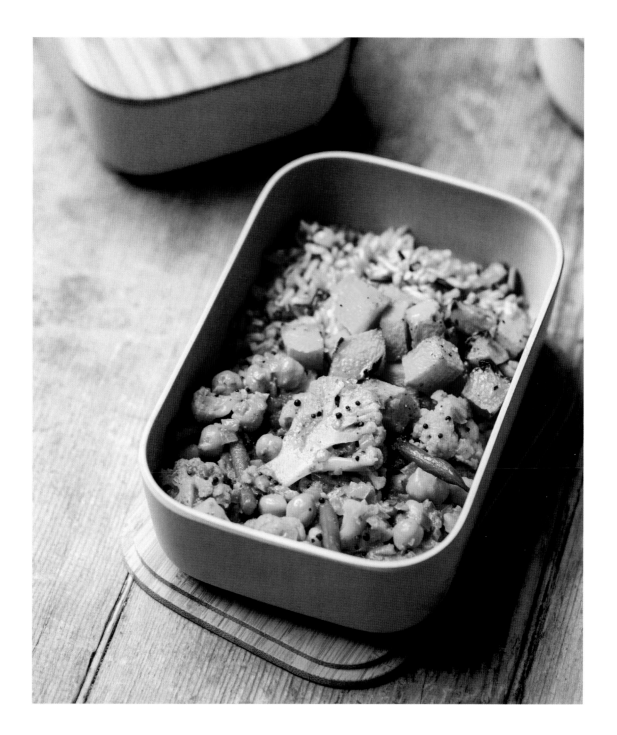

 BONUS The main ingredients in this curry offer a good range of health and performance benefits. Chickpeas are a really good source of plant-based protein, while butternut squash is high in antioxidants and rich in vitamins A and C.

SMOKED PANCETTA AND LENTIL SOUP

This soup has a lovely, hearty depth of flavour from the lentils, and the pancetta enhances the taste and texture. A great healthy lunch to take to work, it's also good to have on standby in the freezer. Serve it with the soda bread rolls overleaf. ❄

SERVES 6

1 tsp vegetable oil
80g pancetta, finely diced into 5mm pieces
1 large onion (100g), chopped
2 carrots, diced (200g prepared weight)
4 celery sticks, diced (150g prepared weight)
4 garlic cloves, finely chopped
2 tbsp thyme leaves
1 bay leaf
1.5 litres fresh chicken stock
400g tin chopped tomatoes
250g red lentils
250g (about ½ head) Chinese leaf cabbage, shredded
A large handful of flat-leaf parsley, roughly chopped
Sea salt and freshly ground black pepper

Per serving: *285 cals*
20g protein   *30g carbs*
8g fat   *7g fibre*

1 Heat the oil in a medium non-stick saucepan over a high heat. Add the pancetta and cook, stirring to colour evenly, for about 2–3 minutes until it has released its fat and turned golden and crispy all over. Remove the pancetta from the pan with a slotted spoon and drain on kitchen paper.

2 Add the onion and carrots to the pan and cook for 5 minutes or until the onion is softened. Add the celery and garlic and cook for a further 3–4 minutes, stirring occasionally.

3 Add the thyme, bay leaf, stock and tomatoes, stir and bring to a gentle simmer. Add the lentils and cook for 20–25 minutes or until they are softened. Remove the bay leaf. Now, using a stick blender, partially blend the soup, keeping a fairly chunky texture.

4 Bring back to a simmer, add the cabbage and cook for 3–4 minutes until it is tender and wilted. Reheat the pancetta in a small pan at the same time if you like.

5 Stir half the parsley through the soup and ladle into warmed bowls or containers. Serve at once, topped with the pancetta and remaining parsley. Or cool, then seal, store in the fridge and eat within 3 days. Reheat until piping hot before serving; finish as above.

TO FREEZE Allow the soup to cool then freeze in one- or two-portion containers. Defrost fully overnight in the fridge, then reheat in a saucepan over a medium heat until hot all the way through. Finish as above, with freshly cooked pancetta and chopped parsley.

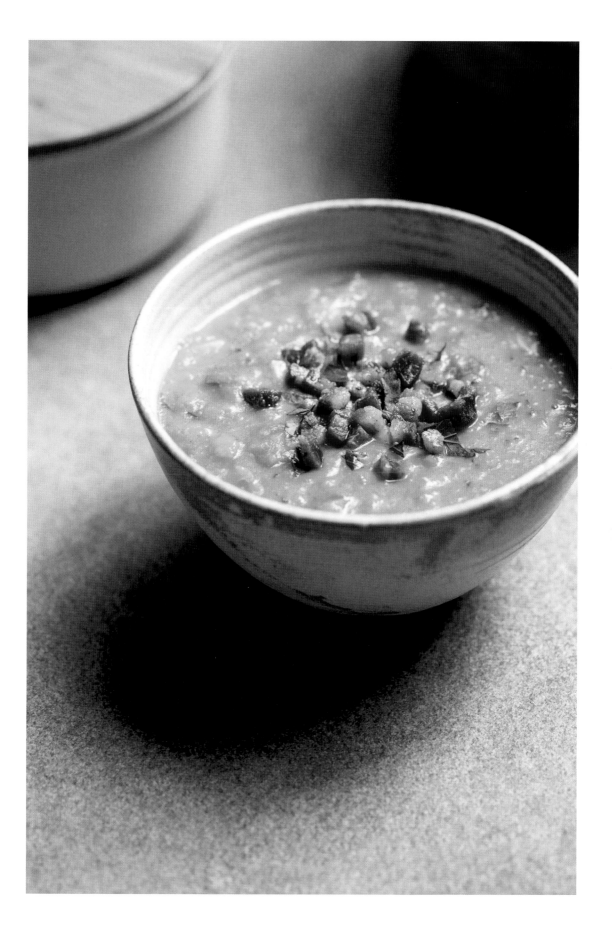

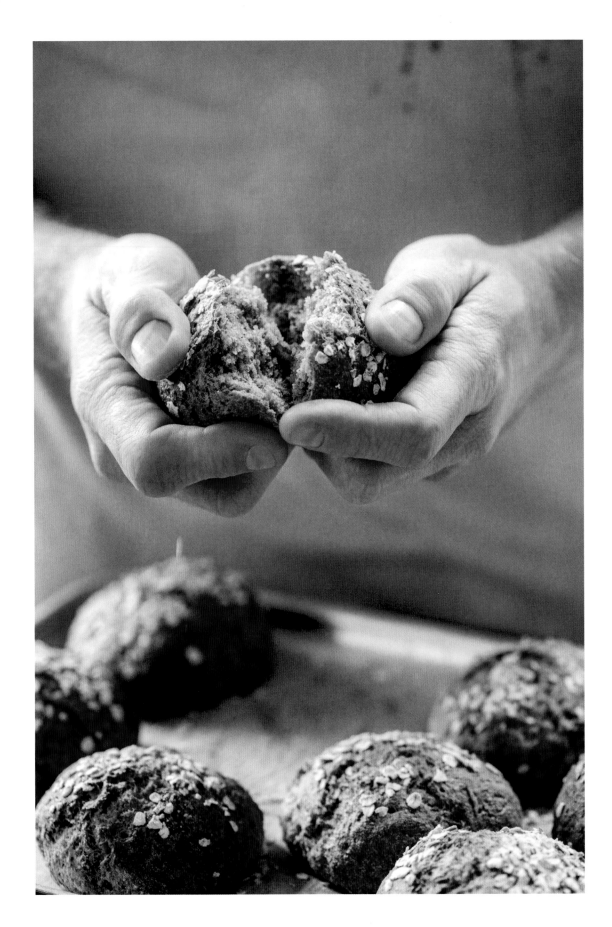

WHOLEMEAL SODA BREAD ROLLS

Easy to make, these rolls are a great way to get into making your own bread. Higher in protein than regular white bread rolls, they have a satisfying full flavour and a fantastic rich colour. The oats on top add an extra layer of texture. Serve them with soups, such as the smoked pancetta and lentil soup on the previous page, and alongside salads or stews. ♡ ❄

MAKES 8

325g wholemeal flour, plus extra for dusting
125g self-raising flour
1 tsp sea salt
2 tsp bicarbonate of soda
1 tbsp soft light brown sugar
250g natural yoghurt
150ml whole milk, plus 1 tbsp for brushing
Juice of ½ lemon
10g porridge oats, for the topping

1 Preheat the oven to 220°C/Fan 200°C/Gas 7. Line a baking tray with a silicone mat or baking paper.

2 Put all the dry ingredients into a large bowl, stir to mix and make a well in the middle. In a jug or another bowl, whisk together the yoghurt, milk and lemon juice, then pour into the dry ingredients. Mix well until a slightly sticky dough forms.

3 Lightly flour your work surface, then tip the dough out onto it and knead gently until smooth. Cut the dough in half and then cut each half into quarters.

4 Roll each piece of dough into a ball and place on the lined mat, leaving a few centimetres between each roll.

5 Brush the tops of the rolls with milk and sprinkle with porridge oats. Bake on a high shelf in the oven for 15–20 minutes or until golden brown and cooked through. Remove from the oven and leave to cool slightly on a wire rack.

6 Serve while still slightly warm, or cool then freeze.

TO FREEZE Allow the cooked rolls to cool then freeze in a ziplock bag or rigid container. Defrost at room temperature then reheat in the oven preheated to 160°C/Fan 140°C/Gas 3 for 5–10 minutes.

Per serving: *244 cals*
9g protein   *45g carbs*
2g fat   *5g fibre*

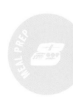

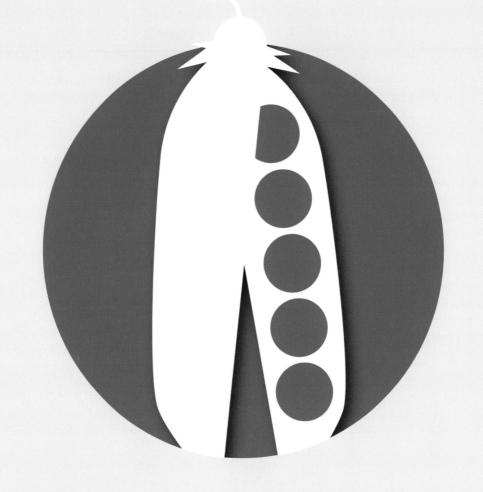

4 MORE VEG

AS A PROFESSIONAL CHEF I'm well known for cooking with meat – and there's no denying I love eating it. That said, I don't think we should see veg as second place. Vegetables are about so much more than simply bulking up a meal or adding a token bit of green on the side. They offer an incredible variety of textures and flavours and they're packed with nutrients, so they can be the stars of the show.

Recently, there's been a big sway towards vegan eating and I think it's great. The fact that it's so big right now will hopefully encourage even the most hardened of meat-eaters to have a few meat-free days each week and enjoy some of the amazing veggies that are available. And as an added bonus, eating more veg will leave you feeling full and satisfied without providing as many calories as meat, which means you can eat more – surely the best news for any dieter!

These recipes all showcase the unique qualities and versatility of different veg. Vegetable dishes can be warming, hearty and comforting as you'll see in my flavour-packed black bean and butternut chilli on page 113, indulgent spinach and ricotta pasta bake (see page 126) and creamy, protein-rich dhal on page 128. Proving that salads can be full of taste and texture and make a satisfying evening meal too, try the warm roast onion, chickpea and halloumi salad on page 122, or beat those burger cravings with a Mexican-style bean burger on page 116. And just look at the incredible colour cavolo nero adds to the pesto on page 114!

There are so many options when it comes to preparing veg-based dishes, that once you decide to cut down on eating meat, you'll actually find you have so much *more* choice for what to eat. As the recipes in this chapter will demonstrate, veg is most definitely not boring.

BAKED RICOTTA-STUFFED MUSHROOMS

The intense flavours of nutmeg, chilli and garlic elevate this simple meal, and the ricotta – a great lower-fat dairy option – provides a luxurious creamy texture. Try to find beautiful big portobellos as they'll hold their shape much better than other large mushrooms. ♥

SERVES 2

4 portobello mushrooms
1 tsp olive oil
1 onion, finely chopped
3 garlic cloves, finely chopped
1 tbsp lemon thyme leaves
50g baby spinach, roughly
    chopped
200g ricotta cheese, drained
A grating of nutmeg
A pinch of dried chilli flakes
4 sun-dried tomatoes, drained
    and finely chopped
1-cal olive oil spray
15g pecorino cheese, finely
    grated
Sea salt and freshly ground
    black pepper

To serve
2 handfuls of rocket leaves
2 lemon wedges

1 Preheat the oven to 220°C/Fan 200°C/Gas 7. Line a baking tray with a silicone mat or baking paper.

2 Carefully remove the stalks from the mushrooms and finely chop them. Place the mushroom caps, cup side up, on the baking tray; set aside.

3 Heat the oil in a medium sauté pan over a medium heat. Add the onion and cook for 3–4 minutes or until softened. Add the mushroom stalks, garlic and thyme and cook for 2–3 minutes. Stir in the spinach and cook briefly until just wilted. Season well with salt and pepper, remove from the heat and leave to cool.

4 Put the ricotta, nutmeg, chilli flakes and sun-dried tomatoes into a large bowl. Add the cooled spinach mixture and stir well. Taste to check the seasoning. Spoon the filling into the mushroom cavities.

5 Spray the mushrooms all over with a few sprays of oil and sprinkle grated pecorino on top of each one. Cook in the oven for 10 minutes and then place under the grill for 2–3 minutes until the cheese is golden brown.

6 Place 2 mushrooms on each plate and add the rocket leaves and lemon wedges. Serve at once.

Per serving: *248 cals*
16g protein   *8g carbs*
16g fat   *3g fibre*

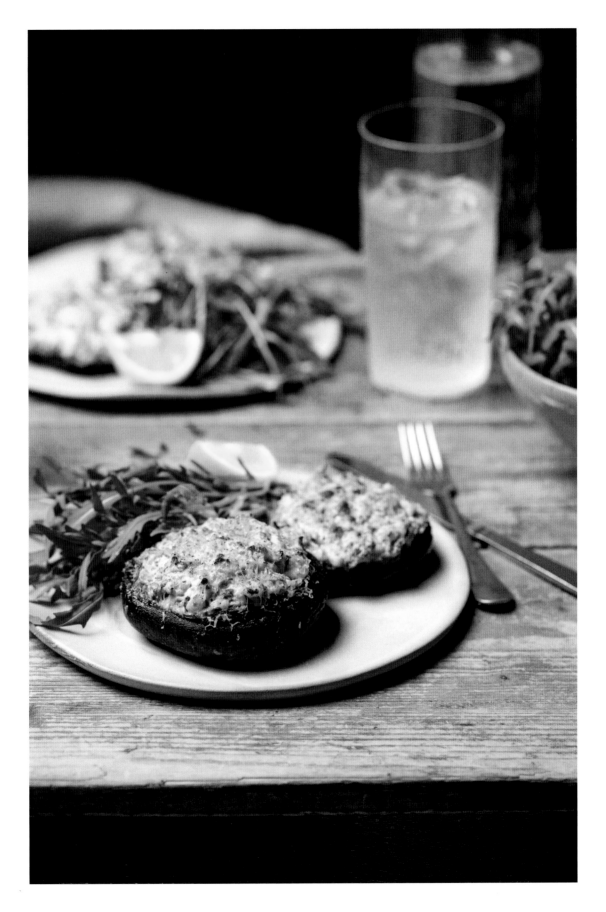

MISO STIR-FRIED GREENS WITH FRIED EGG

 Super-delicious and quick to make, stir-fried greens are a perfect midweek meal when you want to feel like you've really done yourself some good. There are so many flavours going on here, it's hard to believe this dish is as healthy as it is. ♡

SERVES 2

3 tbsp white miso paste
2 tbsp soy sauce
1 tbsp mirin
3–4 tbsp water
½ tsp vegetable oil
½ tsp sesame oil
3 garlic cloves, finely chopped
2.5cm piece fresh ginger, julienned
125g tenderstem broccoli
125g asparagus
125g mangetout
175g cavolo nero, ribs removed and roughly chopped (100g prepared weight)
100g Chinese leaf cabbage, thickly shredded
100g rainbow chard, roughly chopped into thirds
1-cal sunflower oil spray
2 large free-range eggs
1 tsp furikake (Japanese seasoning), to finish

1 In a small bowl, mix the miso paste, soy sauce and mirin with 2 tbsp water until smooth.

2 Place a large non-stick wok over a high heat. When it is almost smoking, add the oils, garlic and ginger and stir-fry for 1–2 minutes, until the garlic is golden – don't let it burn.

3 Add the broccoli and asparagus with 1 tbsp water. Stir-fry for 1 minute, then toss in the mangetout and stir-fry for a further 1 minute. Add a splash more water if the pan looks like it's drying out.

4 Add the cavolo nero, cabbage and miso mixture and stir-fry for 1–2 minutes or until the cabbage is cooked and wilted. Add the chard and cook for another minute, then remove the wok from the heat.

5 Place a medium non-stick frying pan over a high heat. Add a few sprays of oil, crack the eggs into the pan and cook for 2–3 minutes.

6 Divide the greens between warmed plates and top each portion with a fried egg. Sprinkle with furikake to serve.

 BONUS Filled to the brim with vitamins, antioxidants and minerals, greens are particularly rich in nutrients that help reduce muscle aches after exercising.

Per serving: *276 cals*
21g protein   *20g carbs*
11g fat   *9g fibre*

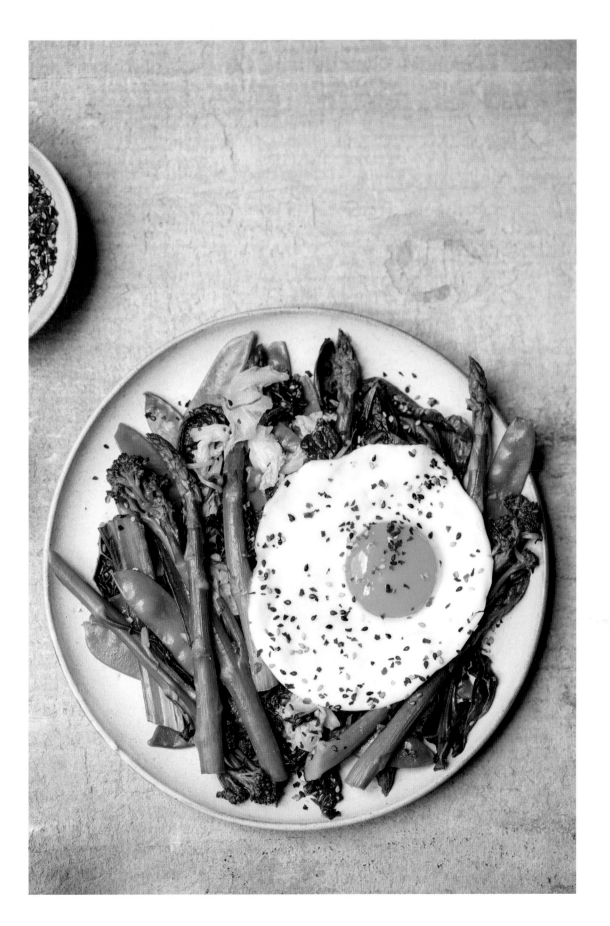

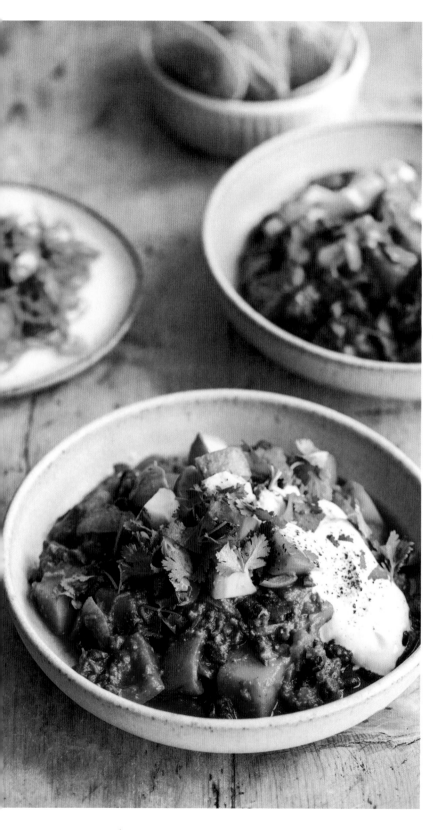
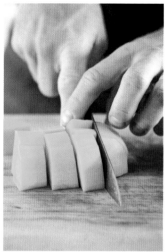
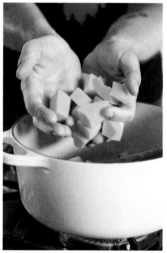
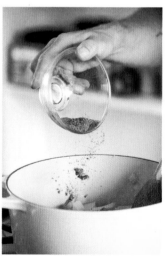

BLACK BEAN AND BUTTERNUT CHILLI

This is the kind of meal to serve the diehard meat-eaters in your life. The powerful smoky Mexican tastes are so amazing they won't miss the meat in this flavour-packed chilli. ♡ ❄

SERVES 4

700g peeled, deseeded
    butternut squash
1 tbsp olive oil
1 onion, diced
3 garlic cloves, finely chopped
2 tsp ground cumin
1 tsp paprika
1 tsp dried oregano
1 tbsp chipotle paste
500ml fresh vegetable stock
400g tin chopped tomatoes
1 red pepper, cored, deseeded
    and cut into large dice
1 green pepper, cored,
    deseeded and cut into large
    dice
2 x 400g tins black beans,
    drained (470g total
    drained weight)

To finish and serve
1 ripe avocado
2 spring onions
2 large handfuls of coriander
    leaves, roughly chopped
4 tbsp reduced-fat soured
    cream
100g tortilla chips

1 Cut the butternut squash into 2.5cm chunks. Heat the oil in a large non-stick saucepan over a medium-high heat. Add the onion and cook for 3–4 minutes until softened. Add the garlic and squash and cook for 2–3 minutes.

2 Sprinkle in the cumin and paprika, stir well and cook for 1 minute. Add the oregano, chipotle paste, stock and tomatoes, stir again and bring to a simmer. Cook for 10 minutes.

3 Add the diced peppers and black beans to the pan. Put the lid on and cook for 15–20 minutes or until the squash is tender and the sauce is thickened.

4 In the meantime, halve, stone and peel the avocado, then dice the flesh. Finely slice the spring onions on an angle.

5 Stir half the coriander through the chilli and divide between warmed bowls. Top each portion with a dollop of soured cream, diced avocado, spring onions and the remaining coriander. Grind over some pepper and serve tortilla chips on the side for crunch.

TO FREEZE Let cool, then freeze in one- or two-portion containers. Defrost overnight in the fridge, then reheat in the microwave or in a pan over a medium heat, stirring occasionally, until hot right through.

Per serving: *553 cals*
18g protein   *64g carbs*
21g fat   *19g fibre*

BONUS If you are looking to have a lower-calorie meal, you can still enjoy this chilli. Leaving off the soured cream and tortilla chips will save you 147 calories.

CAVOLO NERO PENNE

Cavolo nero is probably my all-time favourite leafy veg – it's like cabbage on steroids with its punchy, irony flavour. In this quick and easy dish, it's made into a pesto and mixed through pasta. Just look at that amazing colour! ♡

SERVES 2

400ml fresh vegetable stock
3 garlic cloves, sliced
280g cavolo nero, stems removed (150g prepared weight)
200g wholewheat penne
20ml extra-virgin olive oil
25g Parmesan, grated
2 tbsp reduced-fat cream cheese
10g toasted pine nuts
Sea salt and freshly ground black pepper

1 Place a large, deep frying pan over a high heat. Pour in the stock and bring to the boil. Add the garlic. Tear the cavolo leaves in half, add to the pan and press down with the back of a spoon to submerge them in the stock. Cook for 4–5 minutes.

2 Meanwhile, half-fill a medium saucepan with boiling water and season well with salt. (You want just enough water to cover the penne to ensure that the cooking water will be as starchy as possible.) Add the pasta, stir well and cook until it is only just *al dente* (aim for a couple of minutes less than the packet suggested cooking time).

3 Scoop the cooked cavolo nero and garlic out of the stock and place in a food processor with a little of the stock. Add the extra-virgin olive oil, 20g Parmesan and a little salt and pepper. Blend until smooth.

4 Drain the pasta, saving the water. Add a ladleful of the pasta water to the pan containing the stock and bring to a simmer over a high heat. Add the cavolo nero pesto and the cooked pasta to the pan. Stir well and add enough of the saved pasta water to create a sauce. Stir in the cream cheese until melted.

5 Serve in warmed bowls, sprinkled with the remaining Parmesan and the toasted pine nuts.

Per serving: *574 cals*
24g protein   *68g carbs*
20g fat   *15g fibre*

BONUS Wholewheat pasta contains twice as much fibre as regular pasta – keeping you feeling fuller for longer after eating.

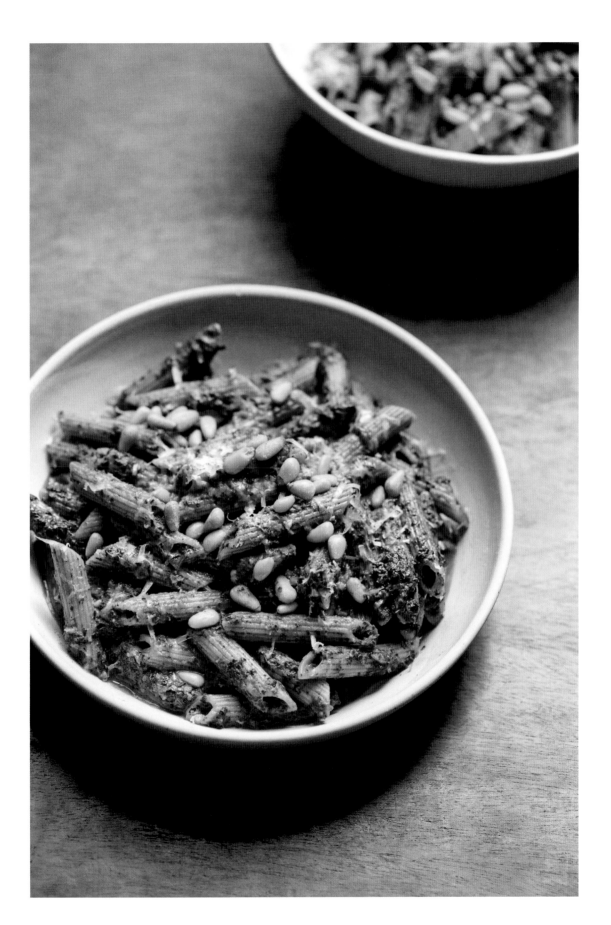

SPICY MEXICAN-STYLE BEAN BURGER

This veggie burger really delivers on flavour and texture – it's delicious. For less heat, leave out the pickled jalapeños. ♡ ❄

SERVES 4

2 tsp olive oil
1 onion, diced
2 garlic cloves, finely chopped
1 red pepper, cored, deseeded and diced
2 fresh green jalapeño peppers, deseeded and finely chopped
1 tsp ground cumin
1 tsp sweet smoked paprika
400g tin red kidney beans, drained and rinsed (240g drained weight)
250g cooked Puy lentils (freshly cooked and drained or a pouch)
1-cal olive oil spray
Sea salt and freshly ground black pepper

To serve

100ml reduced-fat soured cream
2 tsp chipotle in adobo
4 wholemeal burger buns, split
2 medium tomatoes, thickly sliced
1 ripe avocado, halved, peeled and thinly sliced
12 pickled jalapeño peppers
8–12 Little Gem lettuce leaves

Per serving: *445 cals*
20g protein   *51g carbs*
15g fat   *16g fibre*

1 Heat the oil in a non-stick medium frying pan over a high heat. Add the onion and cook for 4 minutes to soften. Add the garlic and cook for 2 minutes. Add the red pepper and fresh jalapeños and cook for a further 2 minutes. Stir in the spices, season generously with salt and cook for a further minute. Take off the heat.

2 Pat the kidney beans dry then tip them into a food processor and add the onion mix. Pulse to combine, retaining some texture. Transfer to a large bowl and mix in the lentils and some salt and pepper.

3 With wet hands, to prevent sticking, divide the mixture into 4 equal portions and shape into patties. Lay them on a plate and chill in the fridge for 30 minutes. Preheat the oven to 200°C/Fan 180°C/Gas 6.

4 Heat a medium non-stick frying pan over a high heat and spray the surface with oil. Add the patties and cook for 2 minutes on each side, spraying with a little more oil before you turn them. Transfer the patties to a baking tray and cook in the oven for 10 minutes.

5 In the meantime, mix the soured cream and chipotle together. Place the burger buns, cut side up, under a hot grill for 1–2 minutes until lightly toasted. Spread each side of the burger buns with chipotle soured cream. Place the bean burgers on the bottom half and top with tomato, avocado, jalapeños and lettuce. Sandwich together with the bun lids to serve.

TO FREEZE Freeze the chilled uncooked patties on a tray until firm, then pack in a ziplock bag interleaved with greaseproof paper. Defrost fully overnight in the fridge, then cook as per the recipe.

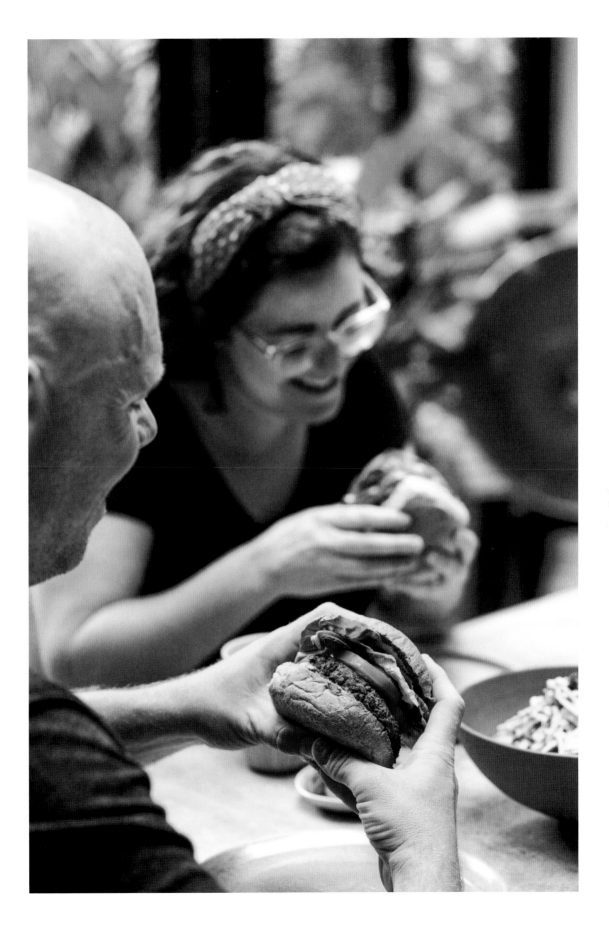

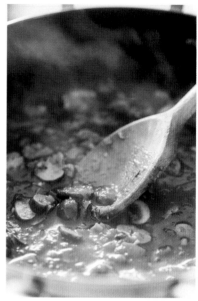

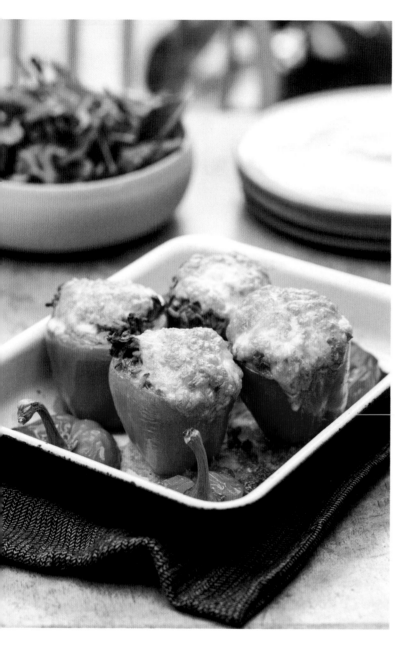

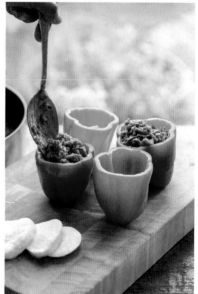

ROASTED MUSHROOM-STUFFED PEPPERS

Truffle paste and dried mushrooms add a wonderful depth and richness to this hearty dish. The delicious gooeyness of the melted mozzarella is an added bonus – providing an extra layer of indulgence you wouldn't expect from a lower-calorie meal. ♡

SERVES 4

1 tbsp olive oil
1 onion, finely chopped
2 garlic cloves, finely chopped
250g chestnut mushrooms, sliced
1 tbsp dried porcini powder
90g jar porcini and truffle paste
2 tsp thyme leaves
2 tsp liquid aminos
300ml fresh vegetable stock
250g cooked brown rice (freshly cooked and drained or a pouch)
50ml single cream
10g Parmesan, finely grated
4 large red peppers
100g light mozzarella, cut into 4 even slices
1-cal olive oil spray
Sea salt and freshly ground black pepper
Rocket salad, to serve

1 Preheat the oven to 220°C/Fan 200°C/Gas 7.

2 Heat the oil in a medium sauté pan over a medium-high heat. Add the onion and cook for 4–5 minutes or until softened. Add the garlic and cook for a further 2 minutes, being careful not to let it burn.

3 Add the sliced mushrooms to the pan and cook for 2–3 minutes, adding a splash of the stock if the pan is looking dry. Stir in the dried porcini powder, truffle paste, thyme leaves, liquid aminos and stock. Bring to a simmer and cook for 5 minutes.

4 Add the rice, stir well and cook for 2 minutes. Stir in the cream and Parmesan, then season well with salt and pepper. Cook for 5–7 minutes, stirring occasionally, or until thickened. Take off the heat.

5 Slice the top off each red pepper and scoop out the core and seeds from inside. If you need to, carefully slice off a sliver of the curved base so that they stand upright – be careful not to cut through to the inside.

6 Stand the peppers in a small baking dish and fill them with the mushroom mixture. Lay a slice of mozzarella on top of each pepper. Place the pepper tops in the baking dish alongside and spray them lightly with oil.

7 Roast in the oven for 15–20 minutes or until the peppers are cooked and the mozzarella is melted and turning golden brown. Serve the peppers topped with their lids and the rocket salad on the side.

Per serving: 305 cals
13g protein   32g carbs
12g fat   7g fibre

MORE VEG

ROOT VEGETABLE BOULANGÈRE

Boulangère is one of those classic French dishes that made me fall in love with cooking in the first place. This version is a great veggie sharer to whack in the middle of the table and serve with a big salad. ♡ ❅

SERVES 4

180g carrots (2 medium)
180g parsnip (1 large)
180g potato, King Edward or
    similar (1 large)
180g sweet potato (1 medium)
180g swede (¼–½ swede)
2 banana shallots, finely diced
4 sprigs of thyme, leaves
    stripped
300ml fresh vegetable stock
150ml single cream
2 garlic cloves, grated
Sea salt and freshly ground
    black pepper
Watercress and spinach salad,
    to serve

1 Preheat the oven to 180°C/Fan 160°C/Gas 4.

2 Peel and thinly slice the carrots, parsnip, potato, sweet potato and swede, using a mandoline if you have one, and place in a large bowl. Season very generously with salt and pepper and mix well. Layer the vegetable slices evenly in a 23 x 28cm baking dish, 5cm deep, sprinkling a little shallot and thyme leaves between the layers.

3 Carefully pour over the stock, cover the dish with foil and bake in the oven for 1 hour. Lift off the foil and cook for a further 30 minutes.

4 Meanwhile, pour the cream into a small saucepan and add the garlic and a pinch each of salt and pepper. Bring to a simmer over a medium heat and let bubble to reduce by about half.

5 Pour the hot cream mix over the boulangère and return the dish to the oven for 30 minutes. Remove and leave to stand for a few minutes before serving, with a watercress and spinach salad.

TO FREEZE Allow to cool, then freeze in two-portion foil trays with cardboard lids. Defrost fully in the fridge overnight, remove the lids and reheat in an oven preheated to 200°C/Fan 180°C/Gas 6 for 30 minutes or until hot all the way through. If the surface appears to be browning too quickly, cover loosely with foil.

Per serving: 236 cals
5g protein   31g carbs
9g fat   8g fibre

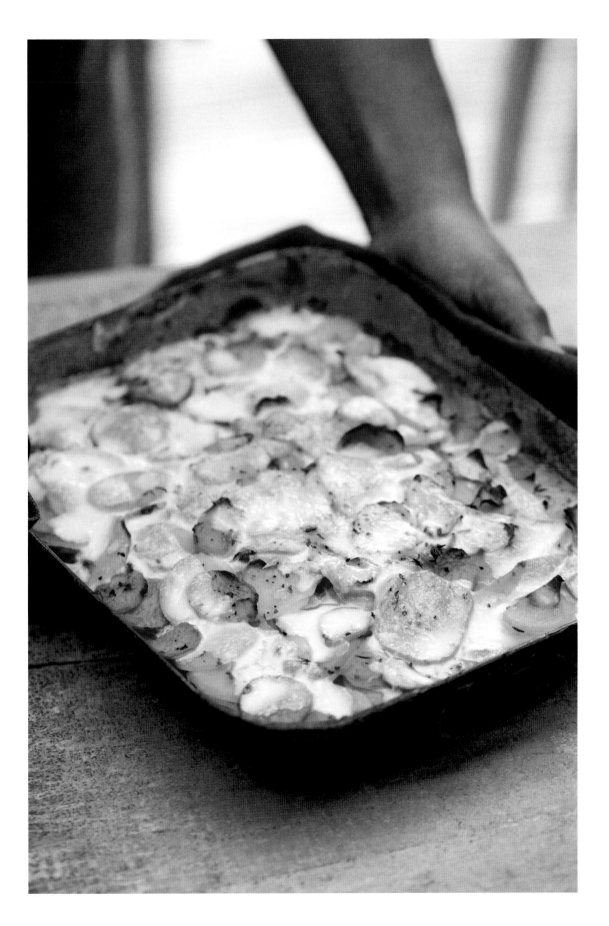

ROAST ONION, CHICKPEA AND HALLOUMI SALAD

Who doesn't love a squeaky cheese?! This warm lentil dish is about as far as you can get from a sad lettuce-leaf salad. Roasting the chickpeas in North African ras el hanout spices gives them an almost crunchy, pub-snack texture once cooked, which works brilliantly next to the springy halloumi. ▽

SERVES 2

2 red onions, peeled
400g tin chickpeas, drained
    and rinsed (240g drained
    weight)
2 tsp ras el hanout
1-cal olive oil spray
250g cooked Puy lentils
    (freshly cooked and drained
    or a pouch)
100g roasted red peppers
    (from a jar), cut into strips
A large handful of mint leaves,
    finely chopped
A large handful of flat-leaf
    parsley leaves, chopped
1 tbsp extra-virgin olive oil
2 tsp pomegranate molasses
125g halloumi, cut into 6 slices
2 tbsp pomegranate seeds
Sea salt and freshly ground
    black pepper

1 Preheat the oven to 220°C/Fan 200°C/Gas 7. Line a baking tray with a silicone mat or baking paper.

2 Cut each of the red onions into 8 wedges and spread them out on the lined baking tray. Add the chickpeas to the tray. Sprinkle over the ras el hanout and a big pinch of salt and rub gently into the onions and chickpeas then spray a few times with oil. Cook in the oven for 20–25 minutes or until the chickpeas are nicely roasted, golden and a bit crunchy.

3 In the meantime, mix the lentils, roasted peppers, mint and half the chopped parsley together in a bowl. Trickle over the extra-virgin olive oil and pomegranate molasses and season well with salt and pepper. Mix well and divide between serving plates.

4 Place a non-stick frying pan over a medium-high heat. Once the pan is hot, spray the surface with a layer of oil and add the halloumi slices. Cook for 2 minutes on each side or until golden brown.

5 Spoon the onions and chickpeas over the lentils, top with the halloumi slices and scatter over the pomegranate seeds and remaining parsley to serve.

Per serving: 685 cals
39g protein   62g carbs
27g fat   20g fibre

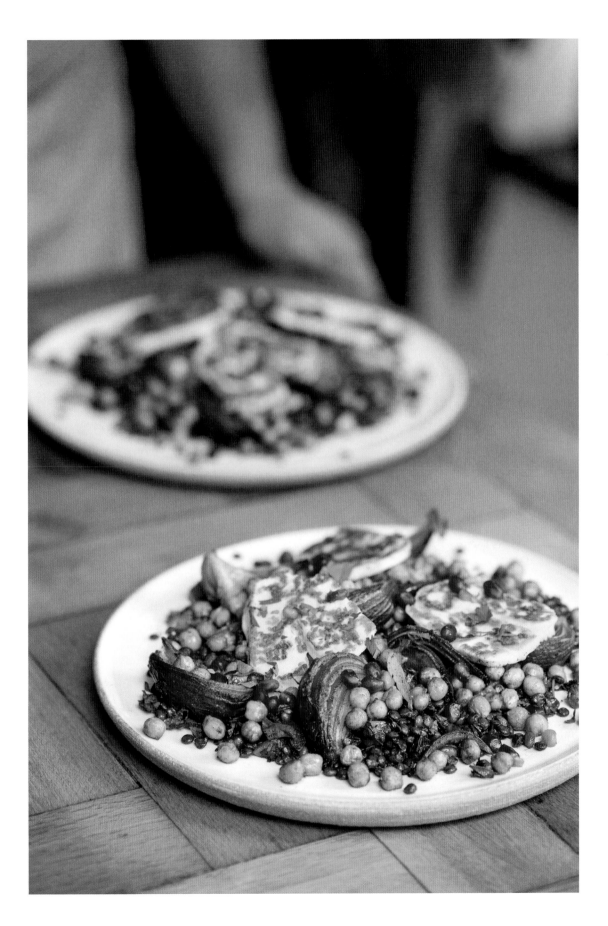

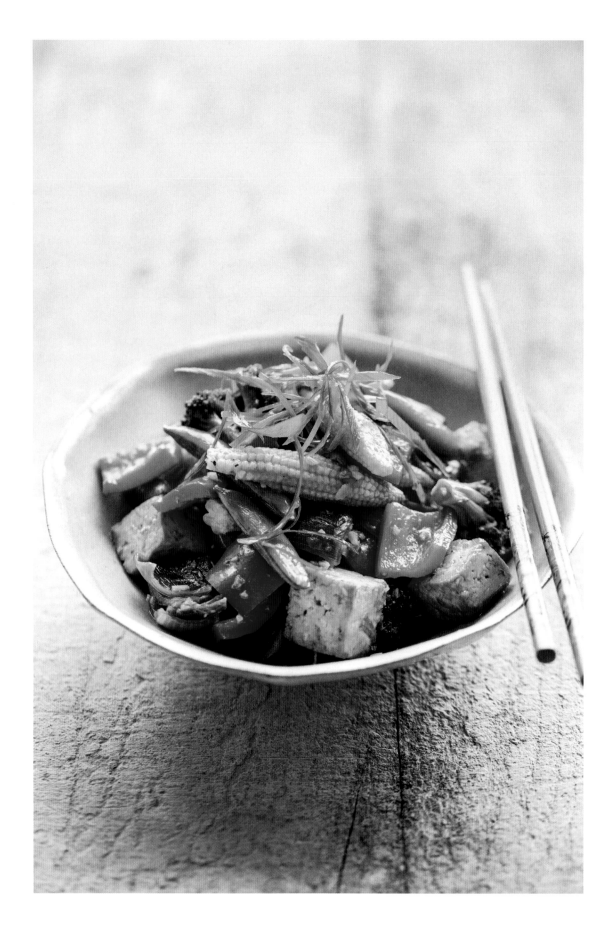

TOFU STIR-FRY

It's no secret that I'm the biggest carnivore out there, so it might surprise you to learn that I really like tofu! Texturally, I think it is brilliant, and it's a real flavour sponge. Give this stir-fry a go and see for yourself.

SERVES 2

1 tsp vegetable oil
1 red onion, diced
225g firm smoked tofu, cut into large dice
2 garlic cloves, finely chopped
2cm piece fresh ginger, finely grated
150g baby corn, cut in half on an angle
200ml fresh vegetable stock
100g broccoli, cut into small florets
1 red pepper, cored, deseeded and cut into large dice
100g sugar snap peas
1 tbsp soy sauce
1 tbsp oyster sauce
1 tsp honey
1 tsp cornflour, mixed with 1 tbsp water
2 spring onions, green part only, finely shredded, to garnish

1 Make sure you have everything prepared and ready before you begin.

2 Heat the oil in a large non-stick wok. When it's hot, add the onion and tofu and stir-fry for 3–4 minutes or until the tofu begins to brown. Add the garlic and ginger and cook for 2 minutes. If the mixture starts to stick at any point, add a splash of water.

3 Add the baby corn and stock and cook for another 2 minutes then add the broccoli and red pepper and stir-fry for a further 1 minute.

4 Add the sugar snap peas to the wok, followed by the soy sauce, oyster sauce and honey. Stir-fry for another 1–2 minutes.

5 Now add the cornflour paste to the wok, stirring as you do so. Cook for 30 seconds or until the sauce is thickened. Serve in warmed bowls, scattered with the spring onions.

BONUS Tofu is a fantastic meat-free source of protein and is low in fat, so it's a great option when you are on a diet. To make this a more substantial meal, serve it with brown rice, allowing 125g each; this will add 200 cals per portion.

Per serving: 376 cals
30g protein   25g carbs
15g fat   9g fibre

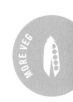

MORE VEG

SPINACH AND RICOTTA PASTA BAKE

A pasta bake is a great recipe to have in your arsenal. This one takes the classic flavour combination of spinach and ricotta and adds the sweetness of roasted peppers and tempting creaminess of melting mozzarella. ♡ ❄

SERVES 6

400g wholewheat penne
1 tbsp vegetable oil
1 onion, finely chopped
6 garlic cloves, finely chopped
1 tsp sweet smoked paprika
250g roasted peppers (from a jar), diced
700g jar passata
400g tin chopped tomatoes
1 tsp dried oregano
100ml water
200g ricotta cheese
A small handful of sage leaves (about 12), finely chopped
150g baby spinach
A handful of basil leaves, roughly chopped
125g light mozzarella, diced
15g Parmesan, finely grated
Sea salt and freshly ground black pepper
Mixed salad, to serve

Per serving: 418 cals
20g protein 59g carbs
10g fat 7g fibre

1 Preheat the oven to 220°C/Fan 200°C/Gas 7.

2 Bring a large saucepan of salted water to the boil over a high heat. Add the penne, stir well and cook, according to the packet instructions, until *al dente*.

3 Meanwhile, set another large pan over a high heat and add the oil. When hot, add the onion and sauté for 4–5 minutes until softened. Add the garlic and cook, stirring, for 2 minutes; add a splash of water if it starts to catch. Stir in the paprika and cook for 1 minute.

4 Add the roasted peppers, passata, tomatoes and oregano. Pour the 100ml water into the passata jar, swirl it around then pour into the pan. Bring to a gentle simmer and cook for 5–10 minutes.

5 Meanwhile, mix the ricotta and chopped sage together in a bowl and season with salt and pepper to taste.

6 Drain the pasta in a colander and rinse under cold running water to cool completely. Drain and set aside.

7 Stir the spinach and basil through the pepper and tomato sauce until wilted. Season with salt and pepper to taste. Add the pasta to the sauce and stir to coat. Transfer the mixture to a large baking dish, about 32 x 28cm and 6–7cm deep, spreading it evenly.

8 Scatter over the diced mozzarella, dot with the ricotta mixture and sprinkle with the grated Parmesan. Bake on a high shelf in the oven for 20–25 minutes. Serve with a bowl of mixed leaves on the side.

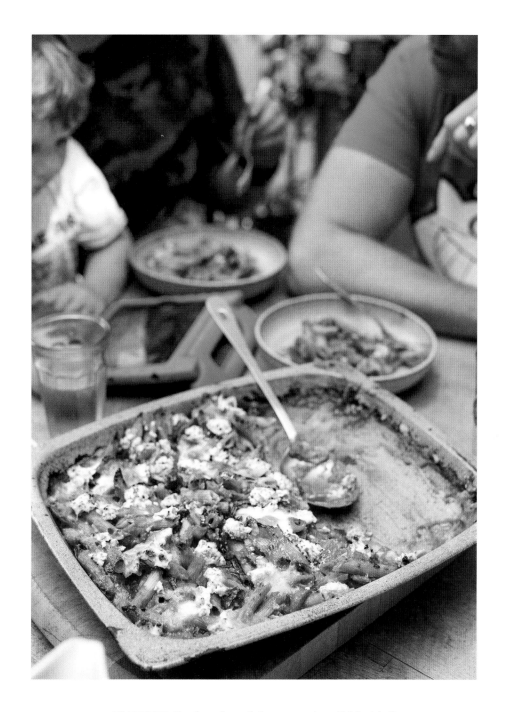

TO FREEZE Cool and pack in one or two lidded foil container(s). Defrost fully in the fridge, then remove the lid(s) and reheat in an oven preheated to 220°C/ Fan 200°C/Gas 7 for 20–25 minutes until hot all the way through. If the surface appears to be browning too quickly, cover loosely with foil.

QUICK BLACK DHAL

Dhal provides a wonderful base for building layers of flavour, as the lentils absorb the spices, garlic and ginger beautifully. If you can't get beluga lentils, feel free to use another type. ♡ ❄

SERVES 4

2 tbsp light vegetable spread
1 onion, finely diced
4 garlic cloves, peeled and finely chopped
2.5cm piece fresh ginger, peeled and grated
1 tsp ground cumin
1 tsp ground coriander
1½ tsp chilli powder
2 tbsp tomato purée
800ml fresh vegetable stock
1kg cooked beluga lentils (freshly cooked and drained or 4 pouches)
100ml single cream
150g baby spinach
Sea salt and freshly ground black pepper
Coriander leaves, roughly chopped, to finish

1 Heat a large sauté pan over a high heat and add the vegetable spread. Once it has melted, add the onion and cook for 6–7 minutes or until it starts to brown.

2 Add the garlic and ginger to the pan, stir well and cook for 2 minutes. Reduce the heat, sprinkle in the spices and cook gently, stirring, for 1 minute. Add the tomato purée and cook, stirring constantly, for 2 minutes.

3 Pour the stock into the pan and bring to a simmer. Add the lentils, bring back to a simmer and cook for 10–15 minutes or until the dhal is thickened slightly. Season with salt and pepper to taste, stir in the cream and cook for 2–3 minutes.

4 Add the baby spinach to the pan, stir well and remove the pan from the heat. Serve the dhal in warmed bowls, scattered with coriander.

TO FREEZE Allow the dhal to cool, then freeze in one- or two-portion containers. Defrost fully overnight in the fridge, then reheat in a saucepan over a medium-low heat, stirring occasionally, until piping hot all the way through.

Per serving: *486 cals*
30g protein   *53g carbs*
13g fat   *19g fibre*

128

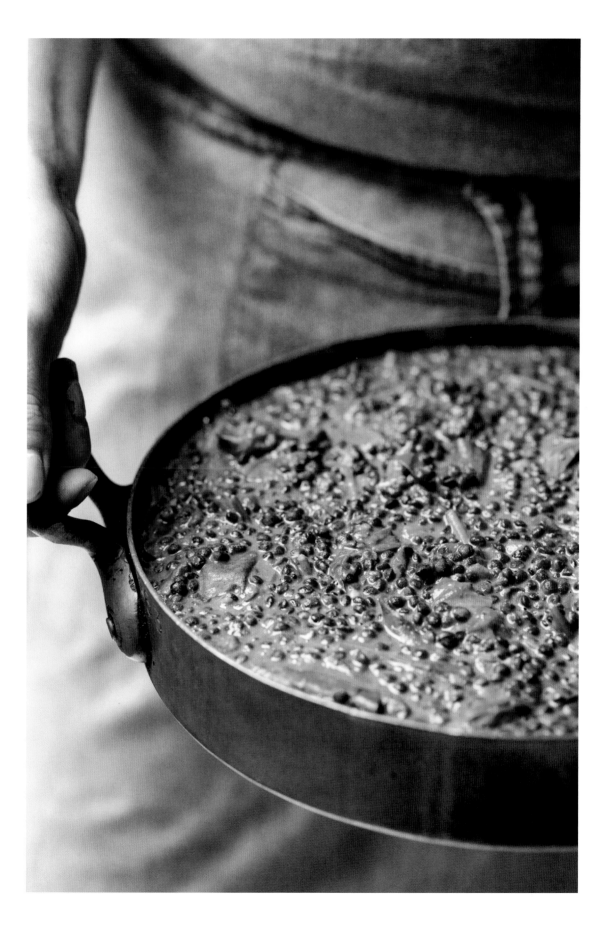

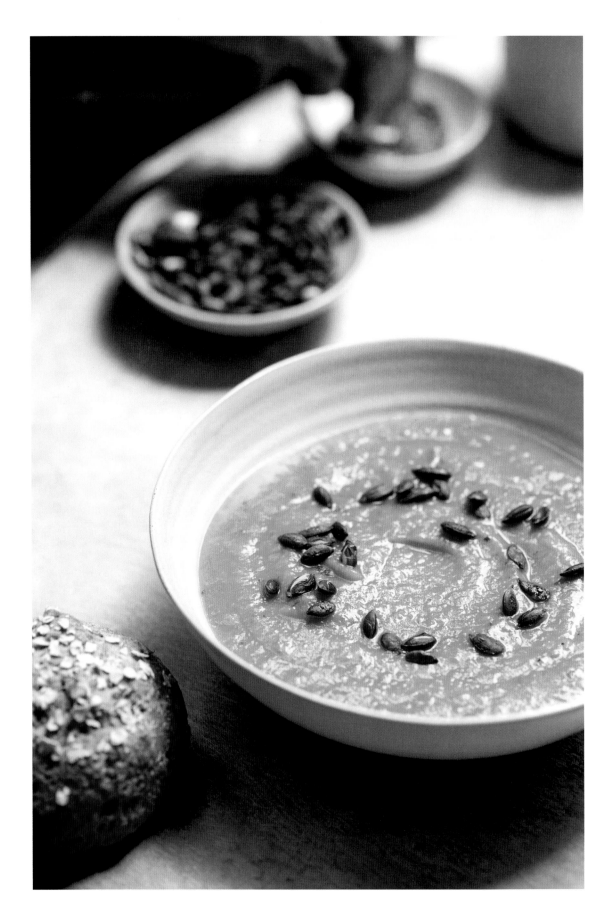

ROAST PUMPKIN AND SWEET POTATO SOUP

A richly flavoured, silky soup made with coconut milk for extra creaminess. Pumpkin and sweet potato are great in soups as they blend really well and produce a lovely smooth texture. ♡ ❄

SERVES 4

500g peeled and deseeded pumpkin, cut into 2cm chunks
500g peeled sweet potato, cut into 2cm chunks
3 onions, halved
12 garlic cloves, skin on
1-cal olive oil spray
1 litre fresh vegetable stock
1 tbsp finely chopped rosemary leaves
1 tbsp thyme leaves
100ml tinned coconut milk
30g pumpkin seeds
1 tsp liquid aminos (or use soy sauce or tamari)
Sea salt and freshly ground black pepper
Soda bread rolls, to serve (see page 105)

1 Preheat the oven to 220°C/Fan 200°C/Gas 7. Line two large trays with silicone mats or baking paper.

2 Spread the pumpkin and sweet potato chunks out on each tray. Cut each onion half into 4 wedges and add these to the trays with the garlic. Season well with salt and pepper and spray each tray a few times with oil. Cook in the oven for 30–35 minutes or until the veg are roasted and tender, tossing them and switching the trays between shelves halfway through cooking.

3 Meanwhile, pour the stock into a large saucepan and add the rosemary, thyme and coconut milk. Bring to a gentle simmer.

4 Place a small frying pan over a high heat. Add the pumpkin seeds and toast until they begin to pop. Remove from the heat, add the liquid aminos and stir to coat the seeds well. Leave to cool.

5 Take the trays of veg from the oven; remove the garlic and set aside. Increase the heat under the pan of stock and tip the veg into the pan. Pop the roasted garlic cloves out of their skins and add them too.

6 Bring the soup to a simmer again and season well with salt and pepper. Blend in a jug blender until fairly smooth. Serve in warmed bowls, sprinkled with pumpkin seeds, with soda bread rolls on the side.

TO FREEZE Allow to cool then freeze in one- or two-portion containers. Defrost fully overnight in the fridge, then reheat in a saucepan over a medium heat until hot all the way through.

Per serving: 281 cals
7g protein   42g carbs
7g fat   10g fibre

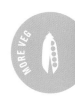

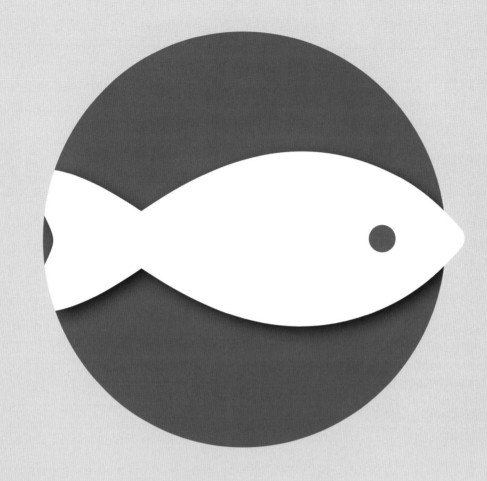

5 FISH & SEAFOOD

FISH IS OFTEN THOUGHT OF as delicate and light, and some people are concerned that it won't fill them up properly – or maybe that it is even a little bit 'too healthy'. However, fish can actually be really robust and meaty, especially if you use a chunky white fish like monkfish, cod or haddock, or a rich, oily fish like salmon or mackerel. It's true that oilier fish contains more calories than white fish or seafood, such as prawns or squid, but it is also rich in omega-3 fatty acids, so it's a really healthy choice.

The recipes in this chapter are all about the flavours. Fish is a major part of people's diet all around the world, and these dishes celebrate ideas from the Mediterranean to Mexico, taking in the Middle East, India and Thailand, as well as good old British fish and chips. If you are not sure whether you like fish, or you're just not used to cooking with it, have a go at some of the spicier dishes first – you'll see just how easy it is to cook and how delicious it can be. Always get your fish and seafood at its freshest – and buy sustainably sourced fish when you can.

Why not start with the tacos on page 134? For this dish, cod is marinated in spices and lime juice, then piled onto tacos and topped with a fresh and fiery salsa; it's all cooled with a chipotle cream. Or on curry night, instead of a takeaway try my creamy monkfish and coconut curry (see page 152); it has a rich sauce that is thickened with lentils, so you don't need loads of high-calorie fats and dairy to make it really tasty and satisfying.

Salmon steaks are a reliable, easy option when you're on a diet – they're quick to cook, you don't need to worry as much about them drying out and they go with pretty much anything. And, although fresh is always best, you can keep some in the freezer for emergencies. Try salmon rubbed with harissa and serve it with an easy lemony-herby couscous (see page 148). Apart from a few fresh herbs you can pick up on the way home (or have a go at growing them on your windowsill), this is a meal you can make in minutes using standby ingredients from your fridge and cupboards. Or flake hot-smoked salmon into a quiche with lots of sweet green veg (see page 156) and have the leftovers for lunch the next day. You can also keep a bag of prawns in the freezer to make saffron rice with prawns and chorizo (see page 147) or the prawn and okra curry (on page 155) in next to no time.

Fish is delicious, versatile and really good for you, so I encourage you to make it a regular part of your weekly menu.

SPICED FISH TACOS

Topped with chunky cod that's been infused with a spicy lime marinade and some crunchy red cabbage, these tacos are finished with chipotle crema and a fresh-tasting tomato salsa with avocado and jalapeño. They'll give you an instant taste of Mexico.

SERVES 2

400g skinless cod loin fillet
6 corn tortillas, 15cm diameter
1-cal sunflower oil spray
200g red and/or white
    cabbage, finely shredded
Sea salt and freshly ground
    black pepper

For the marinade

1 tbsp extra-virgin olive oil
½ tsp dried oregano
½ tsp ground cumin
½ tsp hot smoked paprika
1 garlic clove, grated
Juice of 1 lime

For the chipotle crema

50g reduced-fat soured cream
50g Greek yoghurt (0% fat)
2 tsp chipotle paste

For the tomato salsa

200g cherry tomatoes, halved
1 fresh green jalapeño pepper,
    deseeded and finely diced
A small handful of coriander,
    roughly chopped
1 ripe avocado, halved, peeled,
    stoned and diced
A squeeze of lime juice

Per serving: *670 cals*
49g protein   *50g carbs*
28g fat   *10g fibre*

1 Preheat the oven to 200°C/Fan 180°C/Gas 6.

2 Cut the fish into 12 even-sized pieces and season with salt and pepper. For the marinade, mix the ingredients together in a shallow bowl. Add the fish and turn to coat well. Set aside.

3 Sprinkle a little water over the tortillas, wrap them loosely in foil, place on a baking tray and place in the oven for 5–10 minutes, until warmed through.

4 For the chipotle crema, mix the ingredients together in a small bowl to combine.

5 For the tomato salsa, toss all the ingredients together in a bowl and season with salt and pepper to taste.

6 Heat a large non-stick frying pan over a high heat until smoking hot, then add a few sprays of oil. Now add the fish pieces and cook for 1–2 minutes on one side. Carefully flip them over, trying not to let them break, and cook for another 2 minutes.

7 Spread each warm tortilla with chipotle crema and top with a little shredded cabbage and the cooked fish. Spoon over the tomato and avocado salsa to serve.

NOTE For a striking presentation use blue tortillas, made with naturally blue corn, if you can get hold of them.

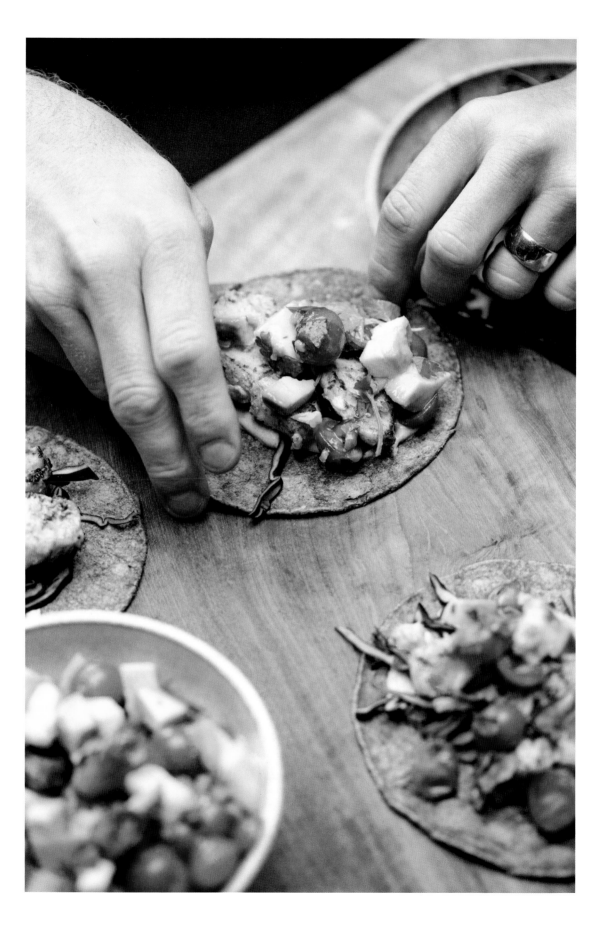

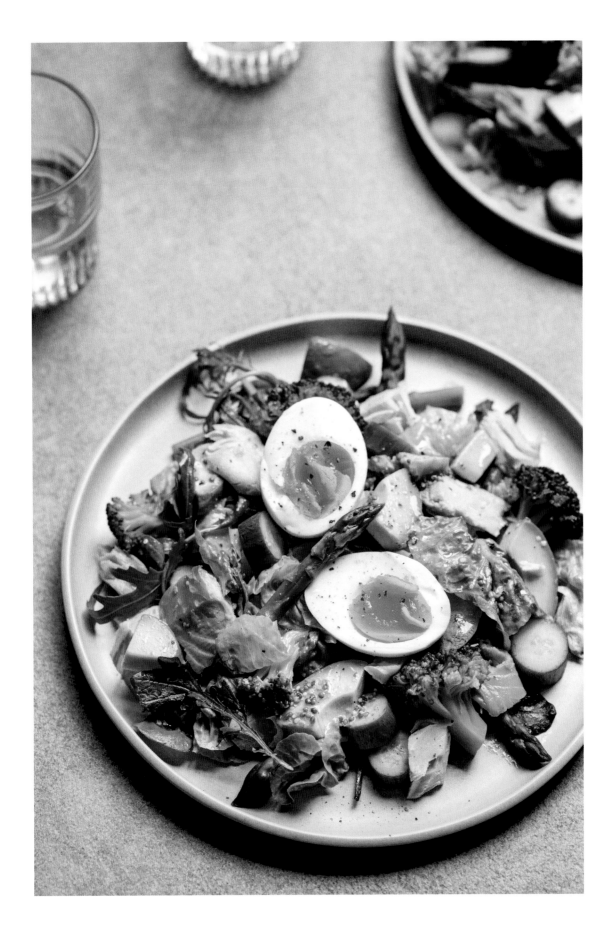

HOT-SMOKED SALMON SALAD

Hot-smoked salmon has a similar smoky flavour to regular smoked salmon but a much more robust texture. You can vary the veg in this salad according to what's in season – courgette or fennel would be great.

SERVES 2

2 large free-range eggs
200g broccoli, divided into
  bite-sized florets
100g fine asparagus spears
  (trimmed weight)
2 Little Gem lettuces
2 handfuls (about 50g) mixed
  salad leaves
2 baby cucumbers, thickly
  sliced
½ ripe avocado, peeled and cut
  into chunks
1½ tbsp extra-virgin olive oil
1 tsp wholegrain mustard
1 tbsp white wine vinegar
A squeeze of lemon juice
150g hot-smoked salmon
Sea salt and freshly ground
  black pepper

1 Bring a medium saucepan of water to the boil over a medium heat and season well with salt. Carefully place the eggs in the boiling water and cook for 4 minutes.

2 Add the broccoli to the pan with the eggs, let the water come back to the boil and cook for 1 minute, then add the asparagus and cook for a further minute. Drain the eggs and veg in a colander, then run cold water over them to cool quickly.

3 Transfer the broccoli and asparagus to a large bowl. Separate the lettuce leaves and cut into bite-sized pieces. Add them to the bowl along with the mixed salad leaves, cucumbers and avocado. Season well with salt and pepper.

4 For the dressing, mix the oil, mustard, wine vinegar and lemon juice together in a separate bowl. Trickle the dressing over the salad and toss gently to coat.

5 Divide the salad between plates and flake over the hot-smoked salmon. Peel the eggs, cut them in half and lay them on top of the salad. Sprinkle the eggs with salt and pepper to serve.

Per serving: *458 cals*
36g protein   *8g carbs*
30g fat   *9g fibre*

FISH & SEAFOOD

CHARRED MACKEREL AND POTATO SALAD

POST

Fresh mackerel tastes fantastic and it's readily available, but people don't cook with it nearly enough. Blow-torching gives it an amazing smoky, charred flavour that goes really well with the natural sweetness of peas and baby potatoes in this salad.

SERVES 2

250g baby potatoes, quartered
80g frozen peas
½ small red onion, finely diced
2 celery sticks, finely diced
2 baby cucumbers, thickly
    sliced
8 radishes, thinly sliced
1 tbsp Dijon mustard
1 tbsp white wine vinegar
2 tbsp extra-virgin olive oil
1 tbsp capers
1 tbsp finely chopped dill
1 tbsp finely chopped chives
Juice of 1 lemon, or to taste
4 very fresh mackerel fillets
    (80g each), pin-boned
2 small cooked beetroot, cut
    into 1cm cubes
Sea salt and freshly ground
    black pepper
Lemon wedges, to serve

1 Put the potatoes into a medium saucepan, cover with cold salted water and bring to the boil over a high heat. Cook for 10 minutes or until the potatoes are tender, adding the peas to the pan for the final minute. Drain the potatoes and peas in a colander.

2 Transfer the warm potatoes and peas to a large bowl. Add the onion, celery, cucumbers and radishes to the bowl. Toss gently to mix.

3 For the dressing, mix the mustard and wine vinegar together in a bowl. Slowly whisk in the oil until the dressing thickens. Stir in the capers and chopped herbs. Add salt, pepper and lemon juice to taste.

4 Line a baking tray with a silicone mat (or spray with a little oil). Pat the mackerel fillets dry with kitchen paper then season both sides with salt and pepper. Place them skin side up on the prepared tray. Run a cook's blowtorch over the skin side until well charred (it doesn't need to be cooked right through, as it can be served rare).

5 Stir the beetroot through the potato salad and divide between plates. Top each portion with a couple of mackerel fillets and serve with lemon wedges.

BONUS Mackerel is packed with healthy omega-3 fatty acids and rich in protein, while beetroot has many health and performance benefits, including lowering blood pressure and boosting stamina.

FISH & SEAFOOD

Per serving: *623 cals*
37g protein   *34g carbs*
36g fat   *9g fibre*

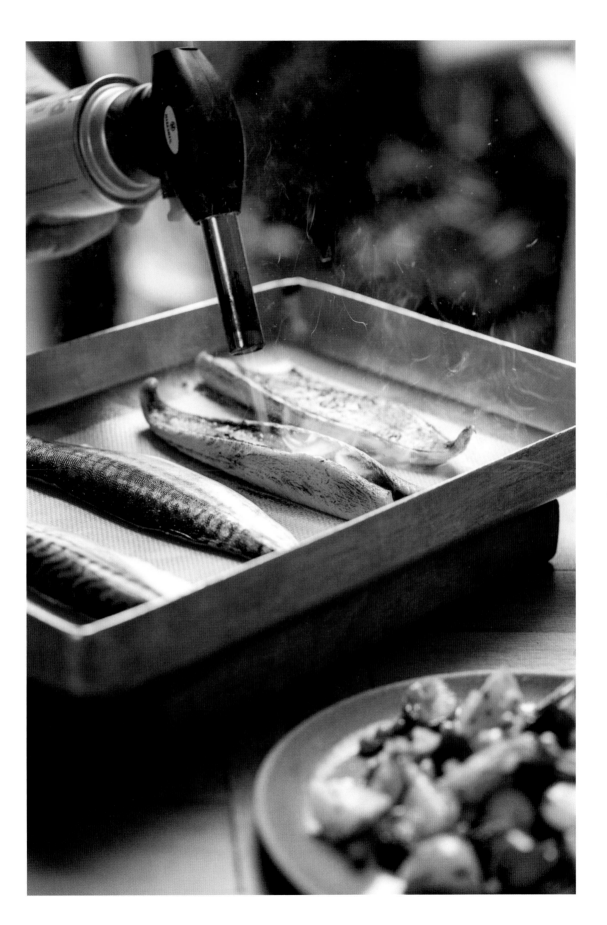

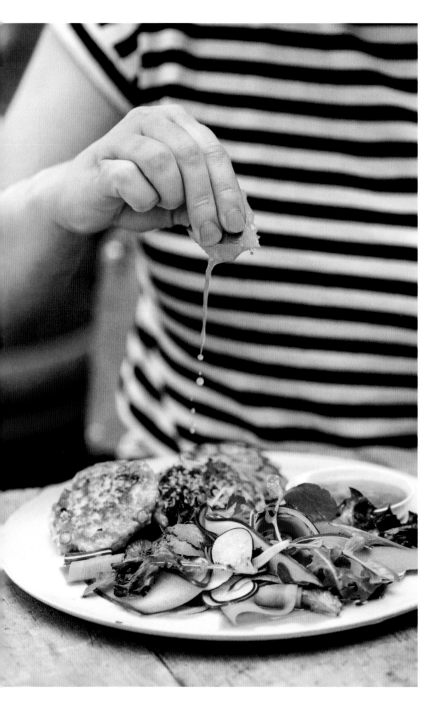

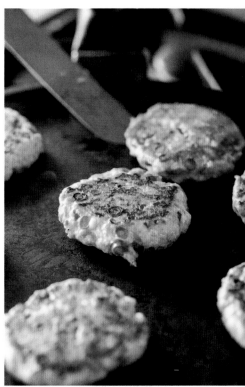

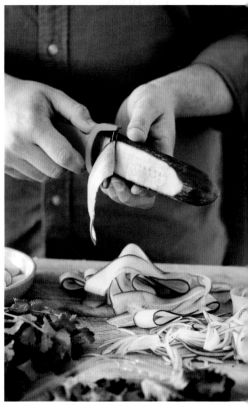

THAI FISH CAKES

Full of intense flavours and with green beans added for extra texture, these fish cakes are easy to make and taste delicious. All they need alongside is a fresh crunchy salad. ❄

SERVES 4

600g skinless salmon fillet
1 large free-range egg
2 tsp lemongrass paste
2 tbsp Thai red curry paste
1 tbsp fish sauce
4 kaffir lime leaves, finely shredded
100g green beans, finely sliced
1-cal sunflower oil spray
Sea salt and freshly ground black pepper

For the salad
2 carrots (200g), peeled
200g cucumber
½ red onion, finely sliced
12 radishes, thinly sliced
A large handful of coriander, roughly chopped
60g mixed salad leaves
1 tbsp rice wine vinegar
1 tbsp soy sauce

To serve
2 limes, halved

Per serving: 354 cals
38g protein   9g carbs
18g fat   5g fibre

1 Cut the salmon fillet into chunks and put into a food processor with the egg, lemongrass paste, curry paste, fish sauce and lime leaves. Season well with salt and pepper and blitz until the mixture comes together, not until completely smooth – leave a few flecks of fish. Transfer it to a bowl and fold through the sliced green beans. Cover and refrigerate until needed.

2 To prepare the salad, pare the carrots and cucumber into ribbons, using a swivel vegetable peeler. Combine with the red onion, radishes, coriander and salad leaves in a large bowl.

3 Place a large non-stick frying pan over a medium-high heat. Divide the fish cake mixture into 8 equal-sized pieces and shape into patties – you'll need to cook them in batches. Spray a little oil into the pan and add half of the fish cakes, spacing them well apart and flattening each one slightly. Cook for 2–3 minutes on each side.

4 Add the rice vinegar and soy sauce to the salad and mix well. Taste to check the seasoning, adding salt and pepper if needed.

5 Divide the salad between serving plates and add 2 fish cakes and a lime half to each plate. Serve with a little sweet chilli dipping sauce if you like.

TO FREEZE Place the uncooked patties on a tray lined with greaseproof paper or a silicone mat and freeze until firm, then pack in a ziplock bag. Defrost fully in the fridge before cooking as per the recipe.

FISH & SEAFOOD

141

OVEN-BAKED FISH FINGERS

A posh way of doing a childhood favourite! The crumb coating for the fish fingers includes herbs and garlic for extra flavour, but you could leave the garlic out if you're making them for kids who don't like it. Everyone will love the baked sweet potato wedges.

SERVES 2

2 small sweet potatoes, cut into wedges (350g prepared weight)
½ tsp sweet smoked paprika
1-cal sunflower oil spray
350g skinless cod loin or haddock fillet
20g dried onion flakes
1 tsp garlic granules
1 tbsp finely chopped fresh rosemary
Grated zest of 1 lemon
20g panko breadcrumbs
1 large free-range egg white
Sea salt and freshly ground black pepper

For the minted peas
100g frozen peas
1 tbsp light vegetable spread
1 tbsp finely chopped mint

For the tartare sauce
2 tbsp light mayonnaise
2 tbsp Greek yoghurt (0% fat)
3 cornichons, finely chopped
1 tsp baby capers
1 tsp Dijon mustard
1 tbsp finely chopped flat-leaf parsley
Lemon juice, to taste

To serve
Lemon wedges

1 Preheat the oven to 230°C/Fan 220°C/Gas 8. Line 2 baking trays with silicone mats or baking paper.

2 Lay the sweet potato wedges on one of the trays. Sprinkle with paprika, salt and pepper, and spray with oil. Roast on the top shelf of the oven for 25 minutes, checking the potatoes from time to time as they cook and spraying with more oil if you think they need it.

3 Meanwhile, cut the fish fillet into 6 even-sized fish finger portions and season with salt and pepper.

4 Grind the onion flakes in a mini food processor. Tip into a shallow bowl, add the garlic granules, rosemary, lemon zest, breadcrumbs and some salt and pepper. Mix well. In another shallow bowl, use a fork to whisk the egg white with some salt and pepper.

5 Dip each piece of fish into the egg white and then into the crumbs to coat completely. Place on the other lined baking tray and spray liberally with oil.

6 Move the sweet potatoes to the middle oven shelf and place the tray of fish fingers on the top shelf. Cook for 8–10 minutes or until golden. There's no need to turn the fish fingers – if the crumb coating isn't browned enough, place under the grill for a minute or two.

7 While the fish fingers are cooking, put the peas into a small saucepan with the vegetable spread and mint. Cook over a medium heat for 2–3 minutes with the lid on. Season the peas with salt and pepper to taste and mash them lightly.

FISH & SEAFOOD

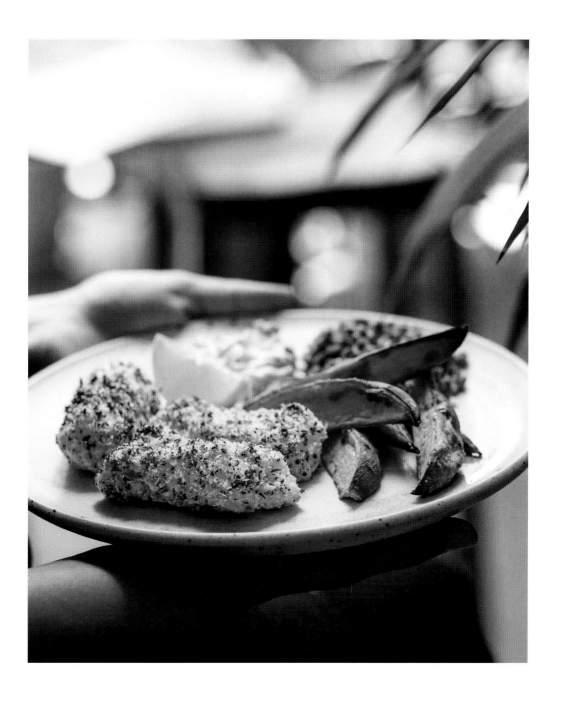

8 For the tartare sauce, mix the ingredients together in a small bowl and season with salt and pepper to taste.

Per serving: *480 cals*
42g protein   *51g carbs*
10g fat   *9g fibre*

9 Take the sweet potato wedges and fish fingers out of the oven. Serve on warmed plates with the minted peas, tartare sauce and lemon wedges.

ROAST SALMON WITH PEA PESTO

This pesto is absolutely packed with flavour from all the fresh herbs, while the peas add a lovely sweetness. It goes really well with new potatoes and cuts through the richness of the salmon.

SERVES 6

500g baby new potatoes
1-cal sunflower oil spray
2 fennel bulbs, tough outer layer removed (600g prepared weight)
Juice of 1 lemon
1kg skinless salmon fillet
Sea salt and freshly ground black pepper

For the pea pesto
3 tbsp olive oil
1 tbsp Dijon mustard
2 tbsp red wine vinegar
2 tbsp water
2 handfuls of basil leaves
A handful of mint leaves
A handful of flat-leaf parsley
300g frozen peas, defrosted
1 banana shallot, finely diced
2 tbsp finely chopped chives
2 tbsp finely chopped dill
2 tbsp baby capers
2 large handfuls of pea shoots

To serve
1 lemon, cut into 6 wedges

Per serving: *478 cals*
43g protein *20g carbs*
23g fat *8g fibre*

1 Preheat the oven to 220°C/Fan 200°C/Gas 7. Line 2 baking trays with silicone mats or baking paper.

2 Add the potatoes to a saucepan of cold salted water and bring to the boil over a high heat. Cook for 12–15 minutes or until tender. Drain in a colander.

3 Smash each potato with the base of a small pan and place on one of the baking trays. Sprinkle well with salt and pepper and spray with oil. Cook on a high oven shelf for 25 minutes or until golden and crispy.

4 Meanwhile, thinly slice the fennel, using a mandoline if you have one. Spread the fennel slices out on the other lined baking tray. Season with salt and pepper and squeeze over the lemon juice. Lay the salmon fillet on top and sprinkle with salt and pepper. Spray with oil and cook in the oven for 15–20 minutes.

5 Meanwhile, for the pea pesto, in a small bowl whisk together the olive oil, mustard, wine vinegar and water. Put the basil, mint and parsley into a food processor and add the dressing and a sprinkle of salt and pepper. Blitz until the herbs are evenly chopped.

6 Add half of the peas to the processor and pulse until lightly mashed. Transfer the mixture to a small bowl and stir through the remaining peas, shallot, chives, dill and capers. Taste to check the seasoning.

7 Take the trays from the oven and scatter the pea shoots over the salmon and fennel. Serve on warm plates with the roasted new potatoes, pea pesto and lemon wedges alongside.

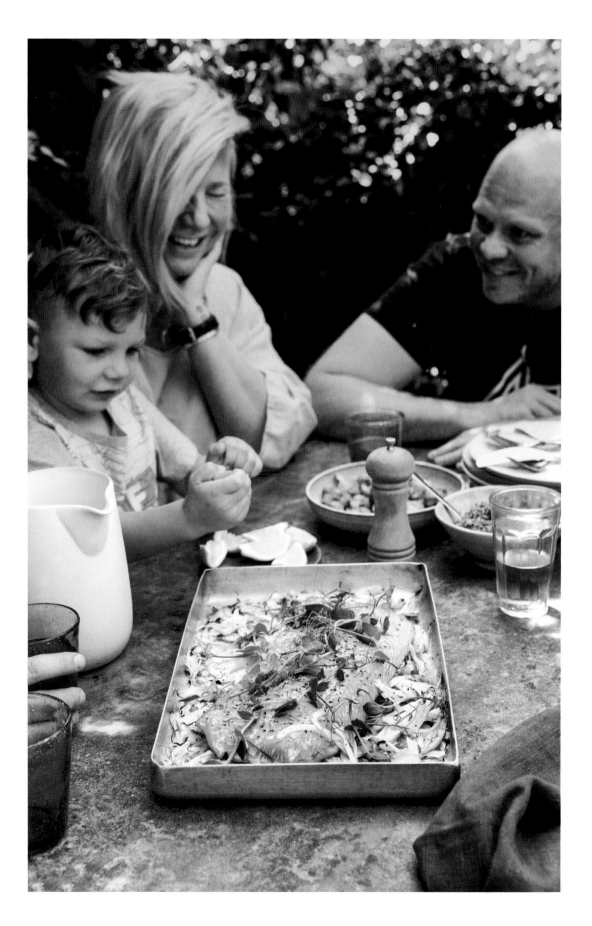

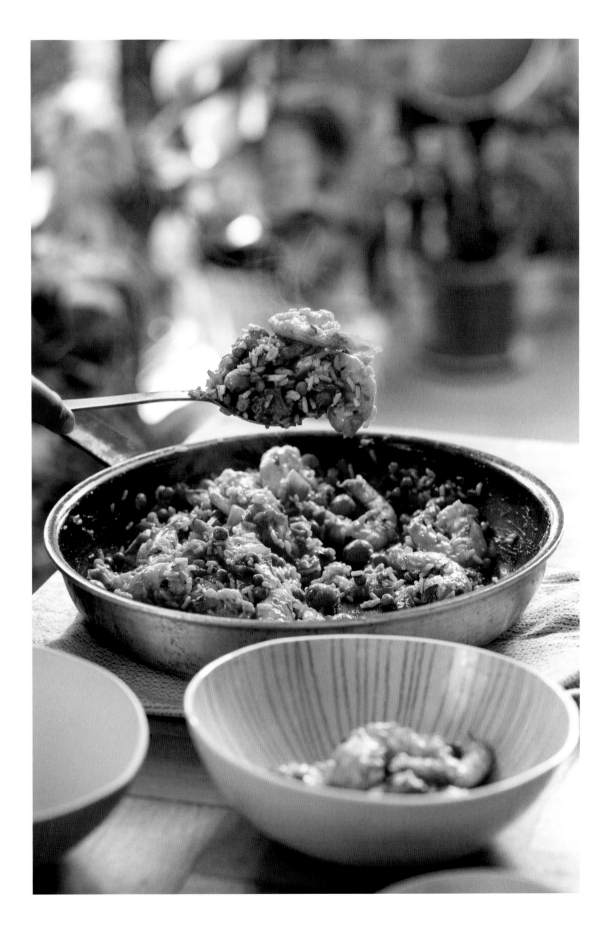

SAFFRON RICE WITH PRAWNS AND CHORIZO

This is my play on a classic Spanish paella. The flavours come from the chorizo and saffron, with the less typical addition of cumin. Piquillo peppers add a subtle acidity and sweetness that perfectly balance the dish and bring it to life.

SERVES 2

1 tsp olive oil
80g spicy cooking chorizo sausage, diced
300g raw tiger prawns, peeled
1 red onion, finely diced
1 large green pepper, cored, deseeded and diced
2 garlic cloves, finely sliced
½ tsp hot smoked paprika
½ tsp ground cumin
1 tbsp tomato purée
A pinch of saffron strands, ground with a pestle and mortar
150ml fresh chicken stock
250g cooked long-grain rice (freshly cooked and drained or a pouch)
100g piquillo peppers, from a jar, roughly chopped
80g frozen peas
50g pitted green olives
1 tsp sherry vinegar
A small handful of flat-leaf parsley, roughly chopped
Sea salt and freshly ground black pepper
Lemon wedges, to serve

1 Place a large sauté pan over a medium heat and add the oil and chorizo. Cook for 2–3 minutes until the chorizo starts to release its oil.

2 Push the chorizo to one side of the pan, then add half the prawns to the other side and cook for 2–3 minutes or until pink all the way through and slightly charred on the outside. Remove the prawns and set aside on a plate. Repeat to cook the remaining prawns.

3 Add the onion to the pan and cook in the chorizo fat for 4–5 minutes to soften, adding a splash of water if it starts to stick. Toss in the green pepper and garlic and cook for 2 minutes.

4 Stir in the paprika, cumin and tomato purée and cook for 1 minute, then add the saffron and stock and bring to a simmer. Now add the rice, piquillo peppers, peas and olives and cook for 2–3 minutes.

5 Return the cooked prawns to the pan and add the sherry vinegar and half the parsley. Stir well and season with salt and pepper to taste. Serve in warmed bowls sprinkled with the remaining parsley and with lemon wedges on the side.

Per serving: *598 cals*
46g protein   *54g carbs*
20g fat   *10g fibre*

HARISSA SALMON WITH LEMON COUSCOUS

Preserved lemons and rose harissa are the stars of the show here. The preserved lemons add a lovely aromatic, citrusy flavour to the couscous and chickpeas, while the rose harissa works like an instant marinade for the salmon.

SERVES 2

80g couscous
A pinch of saffron strands, ground with a pestle and mortar
1 preserved lemon, drained and finely chopped
½ tsp ground cumin
150ml fresh vegetable stock
½ red onion, finely chopped
400g tin chickpeas, drained and rinsed (240g drained weight)
2 baby cucumbers, halved lengthways and thickly sliced
2 tbsp chopped coriander
2 tbsp chopped mint
1 heaped tsp rose harissa
2 lightly smoked salmon fillets, skin on (180g each)
1-cal sunflower spray
Sea salt and freshly ground black pepper
Lemon wedges, to serve

1 Put the couscous into a medium heatproof bowl. Tip the ground saffron into a small saucepan and add the preserved lemon, cumin and stock. Bring to the boil over a high heat, then immediately take off the heat and pour over the couscous. Stir well, cover the bowl with cling film and leave to sit for 5–10 minutes.

2 Preheat the oven to 220°C/Fan 200°C/Gas 7 with the grill element on.

3 Once the couscous has absorbed the liquor and is tender, remove the cling film and fluff it up gently with a fork. Add the red onion, chickpeas, cucumber and chopped herbs. Season with salt and pepper to taste and mix well.

4 Spread the harissa paste over the flesh side of both pieces of salmon. Set an ovenproof non-stick frying pan over a medium heat and spray with oil. Place the salmon, skin side down, in the pan and cook gently for 2–4 minutes until the skin is crispy, then place under the grill to finish cooking for 2–3 minutes.

5 Spoon the couscous onto warmed plates and place the salmon on top. Serve with lemon wedges.

 BONUS Salmon is an excellent source of protein, vitamins and minerals. Here it is combined with couscous and chickpeas, which both release their energy slowly, making this is a perfect recovery meal after a tough workout.

Per serving: *683 cals*
56g protein   *56g carbs*
24g fat   *11g fibre*

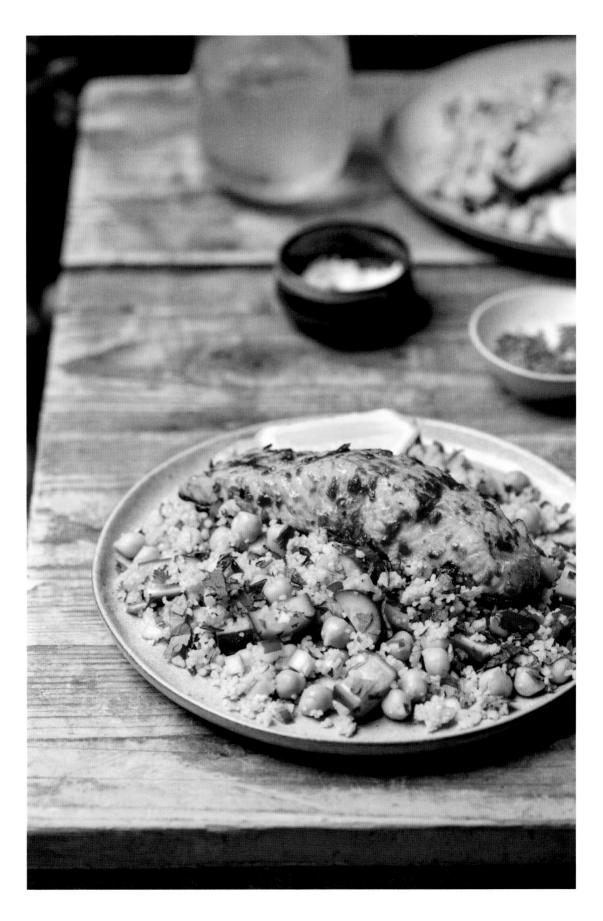

SQUID, CHICKPEA AND CHORIZO STEW

Cooking everything in one pot helps to lock in all the flavours of this Spanish-style stew. Buy the best chorizo you can find as this is where most of the flavour comes from and you're not using a lot. Add an extra pinch of chilli if you like things a bit hotter. ❄

SERVES 2

1 tsp olive oil
80g cooking chorizo sausage, diced
1 onion, diced (100g prepared weight)
2 garlic cloves, thinly sliced
A pinch of dried chilli flakes
½ tsp sweet smoked paprika
1 sprig of rosemary, leaves stripped and finely chopped
50ml red wine
400g tin chopped tomatoes
250ml fresh fish stock
300g medium squid, cleaned
400g tin chickpeas, drained and rinsed (240g drained weight)
50g baby spinach
A small handful of flat-leaf parsley, roughly chopped
1 lemon, for zesting
Sea salt and freshly ground black pepper

Per serving: *543 cals*
46g protein   *32g carbs*
22g fat   *10g fibre*

1 Place a small non-stick sauté pan over a medium-high heat. When hot, add the oil and chorizo and cook for 2–3 minutes until the chorizo releases its oil and begins to turn crispy.

2 Add the onion to the pan and sauté for 2–3 minutes, then add the garlic and sauté for another 2 minutes. Toss in the chilli flakes, paprika and rosemary and cook for 3–4 minutes, adding a splash of water if the mixture starts to stick.

3 Increase the heat to high, add the wine and let it bubble to reduce by half. Add the chopped tomatoes to the pan along with the stock, bring to a simmer and cook for 10 minutes.

4 In the meantime, prepare your squid. Cut the pouches into 4cm pieces, scoring the inner surface, or slice into thick rounds. Cut long tentacles in half.

5 Add the chickpeas to the sauté pan and cook for 3–4 minutes, stirring occasionally. Now add the squid, stir gently to submerge and place a lid on the pan. Leave the squid to cook gently for 3–4 minutes. Season with salt and pepper to taste, remove from the heat and stir through the spinach and half the parsley.

6 Ladle into warmed bowls, grate over a little lemon zest and sprinkle with the remaining parsley to serve.

TO FREEZE Allow to cool then freeze in portions. Defrost fully overnight in the fridge, then reheat in a saucepan over a medium heat until hot all the way through.

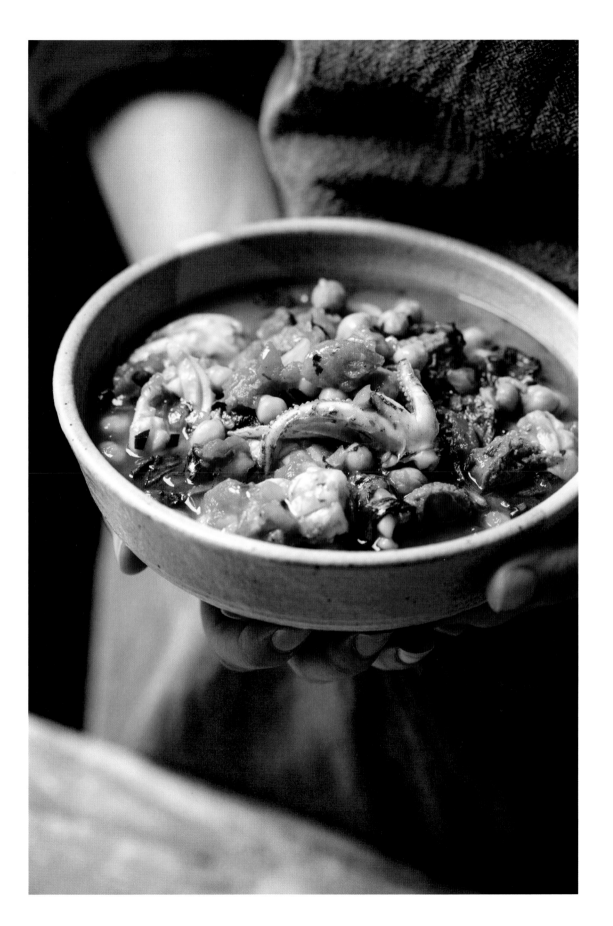

MONKFISH AND COCONUT CURRY

Monkfish is a robust, meaty fish that's great in a curry as it holds its own well with complex spices. Red lentils and coconut provide richness and make this dish feel substantial yet it is still light – the perfect cosy winter feast. ❄

SERVES 2

1 tbsp vegetable oil
1 large onion, finely diced
3 garlic cloves, finely chopped
2.5cm piece fresh ginger, peeled and finely grated
1 long red chilli, finely sliced (with seeds)
A handful of curry leaves
1 heaped tsp ground turmeric
1 tsp ground coriander
2 medium tomatoes, diced
400ml fresh vegetable stock
50g red lentils
400g monkfish fillets
100g green beans
100ml tinned coconut milk
2 tbsp roughly chopped coriander leaves
Sea salt and freshly ground black pepper

1 Heat the oil in a large non-stick sauté pan over a medium-high heat. When hot, add the onion and cook for 5 minutes or until softened and starting to brown.

2 Add the garlic, ginger and chilli and cook for a couple of minutes. Now add the curry leaves, turmeric and ground coriander and cook, stirring for 1 minute or until fragrant.

3 Add the tomatoes, stock and lentils to the pan. Stir, bring to the boil over a medium heat and simmer for 12–15 minutes or until the sauce is thickened and the lentils are tender.

4 Meanwhile, cut the monkfish into 4cm pieces. Trim the green beans and cut them in half.

5 Add the monkfish and coconut milk to the pan and cook over a gentle heat for 2–3 minutes. Add the beans and cook for a further 3–4 minutes. Remove the pan from the heat, taste to check the seasoning and stir in the coriander. Serve in warmed bowls.

TO FREEZE Allow the curry to cool then freeze in portions. Defrost fully overnight in the fridge, then reheat in a saucepan over a medium heat until hot all the way through.

FISH & SEAFOOD

Per serving: 435 cals
41g protein 27g carbs
16g fat 7g fibre

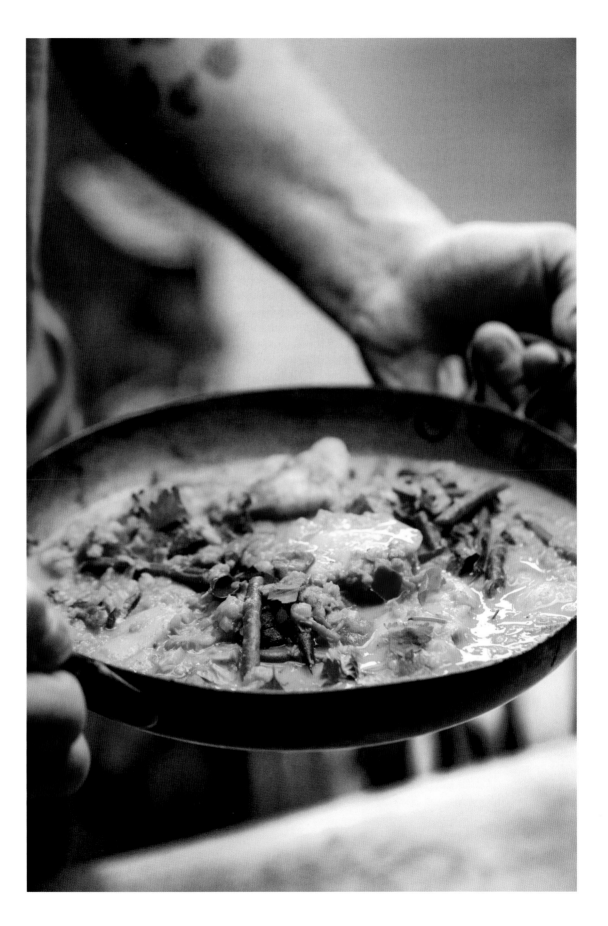

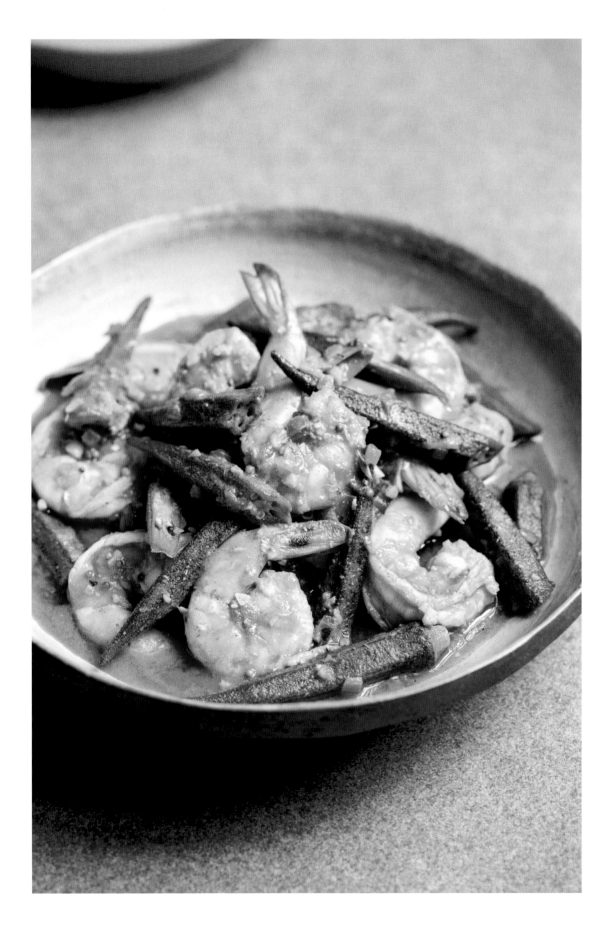

PRAWN AND OKRA CURRY

Okra has a bad reputation for being slimy, but I think that's unfair! Just keep the okra whole and throw it into this prawn curry at the last minute and you'll find it has a good texture. If you can't get tiger prawns, use regular prawns or white fish.

SERVES 2

1 tsp vegetable oil
1 tsp yellow mustard seeds
1 onion, finely chopped
3 garlic cloves, finely chopped
1 tsp paprika
½ tsp hot chilli powder
½ tsp ground cumin
1 tbsp tomato purée
150ml fresh fish stock
100ml tinned coconut milk
200g okra
350g raw tiger prawns, peeled
A small handful of coriander leaves, finely chopped (optional)

To serve
250g cooked wholegrain rice and quinoa (freshly cooked and drained or a pouch)
Lime wedges

1 Heat the oil in a medium non-stick sauté pan over a high heat. When hot, add the mustard seeds and cook until they begin to pop, then add the onion and cook for about 5 minutes until softened and starting to brown.

2 Add the garlic and cook for 2 minutes, then sprinkle in the ground spices and cook, stirring, for a further minute. Stir in the tomato purée and cook for a couple of minutes, stirring regularly. Pour in the stock, stir and simmer until the liquid is reduced by half.

3 Pour in the coconut milk and season with salt and pepper. Simmer gently for 2–3 minutes, then add the okra and cook for 2–3 minutes.

4 Now add the prawns to the sauté pan and cook for 3–4 minutes or until they have turned pink and are cooked through.

5 Meanwhile, if using a pouch of rice and quinoa, heat it up according to the packet instructions.

6 If using coriander, stir it through the curry. Serve in bowls, with the rice and quinoa alongside and lime wedges to squeeze over the top.

BONUS Prawns are a brilliant source of low-fat protein; keep some stashed in the freezer ready to defrost overnight in the fridge before cooking. Okra is rich in vitamin C, which helps muscles to recover after exercise and boosts the immune system.

Per serving: *481 cals*
40g protein   *41g carbs*
16g fat   *10g fibre*

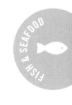

FISH & SEAFOOD

SALMON AND BROCCOLI QUICHE

I love a quiche – hot or cold. Salmon is a great fish to use in a quiche filling as its relatively high fat content means you don't need to worry too much about overcooking it. Wholemeal flour gives the crust a lovely nutty taste and slight crunch.

SERVES 6

For the pastry
200g wholemeal flour, plus a little extra for dusting
1 tsp sea salt
80g light vegetable spread, plus a little extra for greasing the tin
About 80ml cold water

For the filling
150g broccoli
150g asparagus
6 large free-range eggs
100ml whole milk
1 tbsp finely chopped dill
1 tbsp finely chopped basil
250g hot-smoked salmon
100g frozen peas, defrosted
3 spring onions, finely sliced
Sea salt and freshly ground black pepper

Per serving: 363 cals
26g protein   27g carbs
16g fat   6g fibre

1 Lightly grease a 24cm quiche tin, 3cm deep, with vegetable spread.

2 To make the pastry, put the flour, salt and vegetable spread into a food processor and pulse until the mixture resembles breadcrumbs. Add enough water to form a soft dough, pulsing briefly to combine. Take the dough out of the food processor, wrap in cling film and place in the fridge to rest for 15 minutes. Preheat the oven to 200°C/Fan 180°C/Gas 6.

3 Dust your work surface lightly with flour and roll out the pastry on it to the thickness of a £1 coin and 6cm larger than the diameter of your tin. Lay the pastry in the tin, pushing it into the edges and leaving the excess pastry hanging over the edge.

4 Prick the base of the pastry case all over with a fork and line with baking paper. Add a layer of baking beans and bake 'blind' for 15 minutes. Remove from the oven, lift out the paper and beans then return the pastry case to the oven for 10 minutes. Take it out and turn the oven down to 180°C/Fan 160°C/Gas 4.

5 Meanwhile, prepare the filling. Divide the broccoli into small florets, no larger than 2.5cm. Cut the asparagus into 5cm lengths. Place a steamer over a saucepan of boiling water. Add the broccoli and asparagus to the steamer and cook for 5 minutes. Remove the veg from the steamer, drain well and leave to cool.

6 In a bowl, beat the eggs with the milk and herbs and season well with salt and pepper.

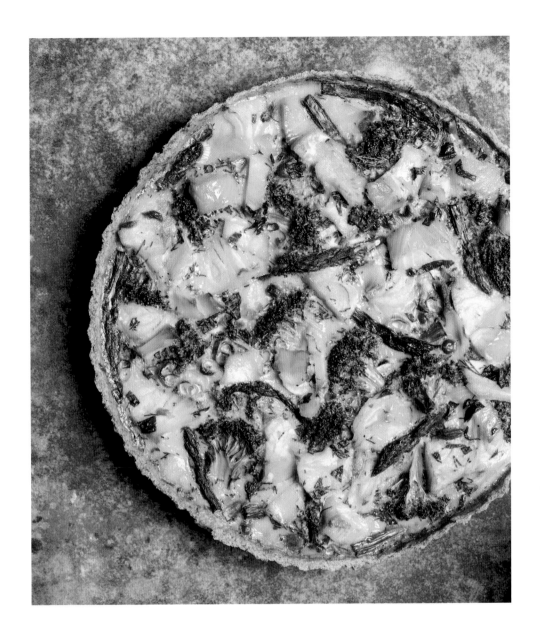

7 Arrange the broccoli and asparagus in the baked pastry case. Flake over the salmon and scatter over the peas and spring onions.

8 Carefully pour the egg mix over the salmon and veg and bake in the oven for 30–35 minutes or until just set. Trim away the excess pastry with a sharp knife.

9 Leave the quiche to cool slightly, then remove from the tin and cut into 6 slices. Enjoy by itself or with a mixed salad on the side.

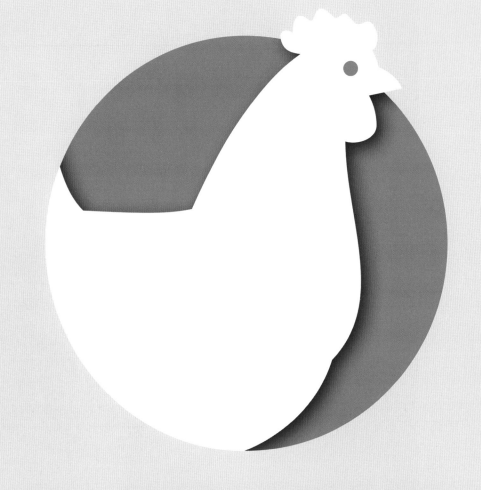

6 CHICKEN & TURKEY

UNLESS YOU'RE VEGETARIAN I think it's a pretty safe bet that you probably eat chicken at least once a week. It's easily available, most people know how to cook it one way or another and it takes on different flavours really well. It is a great choice for weight loss too, as it's a good source of lean protein – especially if you remove the skin. Protein is important when you're on a diet, as it helps you feel full and it also supports your body as it recovers after exercise.

A chicken curry is a classic midweek meal many of us enjoy, and my version on page 176 is super-easy to make, using really tasty, familiar flavours. I think it'll quickly become a regular go-to and a new family favourite. The chicken tagine traybake on page 163 is another great weeknight meal. Traybakes are a real time-saver – you just put everything in a roasting tray and let it do its thing in the oven. It's totally no-hassle cooking, and there's not much washing up either. For something a bit more special, try my Chinese-style chicken pancakes on page 169. These are a healthier version of the ever-popular crispy duck pancakes you come across in Chinese restaurants. And if those cravings for a big, juicy burger get too much, the saffron chicken burger with its delicious harissa yoghurt sauce on page 164 will tick all the right boxes.

I'll also show you how you can take a basic chicken stock and add different flavours to it to totally change the dish. We'll start with a classic Chinese-style chicken noodle soup (on page 170), then head to Vietnam for a traditional pho (see page 173), flavoured with lemongrass and lots of fresh herbs, before landing in Japan to enjoy ramen with soy and miso on page 174. And all three are packed with loads of delicious, crunchy fresh veg. The best thing about these broths is that you can keep portions of the basic stock in the freezer, ready to go whenever you need it.

Turkey is a fantastic low-calorie ingredient, which really comes into its own when it is used as an alternative to minced beef – try it in the meatballs in roasted pepper sauce on page 180 or the hearty sausages and beans on page 186. Both of these dishes are warming, filling meals, but contain far less saturated fat and calories than the regular beef or pork versions.

Keeping to healthy eating for the long term is all about finding dishes and flavours that work for you. Whether it's a curry, stir-fry, salad, traybake or flavour-packed noodle soup, experiment with these chicken and turkey recipes to find your new midweek favourites.

CHICKEN, TOMATO AND MOZZARELLA SALAD

The key to the success of this simple salad is making sure the tomatoes are really ripe and tasty – and to use them at room temperature – don't keep them in the fridge or they'll lose flavour.

SERVES 2

2 skinless boneless chicken
  breasts (180g each)
1 tbsp finely chopped oregano
2 slices Parma ham
1-cal olive oil spray
40g rocket leaves
40g mixed salad leaves
2 Little Gem lettuces (200g
  trimmed weight)
2 ripe tomatoes, sliced
1 tbsp extra-virgin olive oil
1 tbsp balsamic glaze
1 ball (125g) light mozzarella
Sea salt and freshly ground
  black pepper
A large handful of basil leaves,
  to finish

1 Place each chicken breast between 2 sheets of cling film. Using a rolling pin, lightly pound the thicker areas so the chicken breasts are an even thickness (about 2cm).

2 Sprinkle both sides of the chicken with salt, pepper and oregano. Wrap each chicken breast in a slice of Parma ham.

3 Place a large non-stick griddle pan over a medium-high heat. Spray the chicken a few times with olive oil. When the griddle is hot, lay the chicken breasts on it and cook for 3–4 minutes on each side, pressing them down as they cook to ensure good contact with the pan.

4 In the meantime, put the rocket and mixed salad leaves into a large bowl. Separate the lettuce leaves, tear into bite-sized pieces and add to the bowl, with the tomatoes. Sprinkle with a little salt and pepper, add the olive oil and balsamic glaze and toss gently.

5 Divide the salad between serving plates. Tear the mozzarella into pieces and scatter over the salad. Season with salt and pepper to taste and top with the chicken. Finish with a scattering of basil leaves.

Per serving: *359 cals*
45g protein *7g carbs*
16g fat *3g fibre*

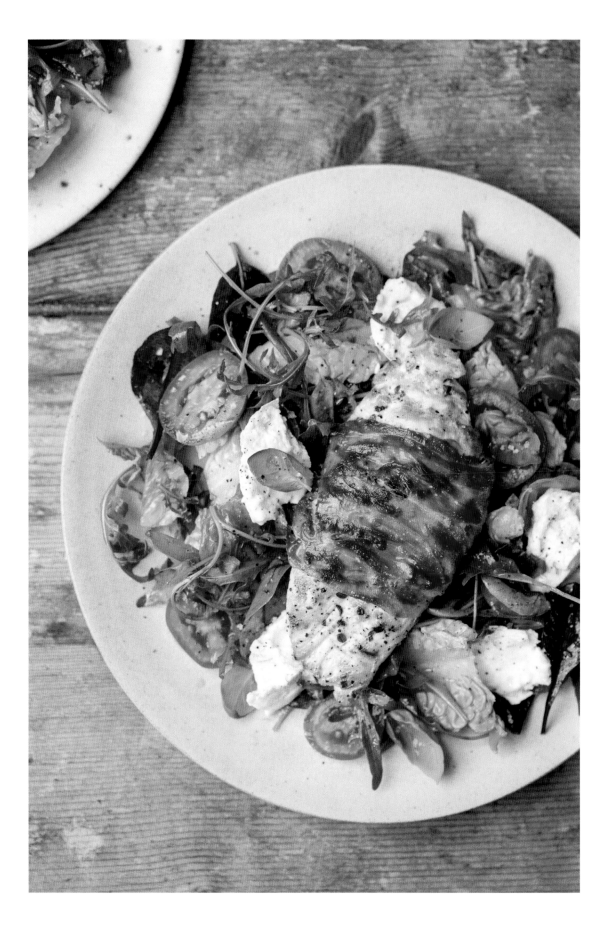

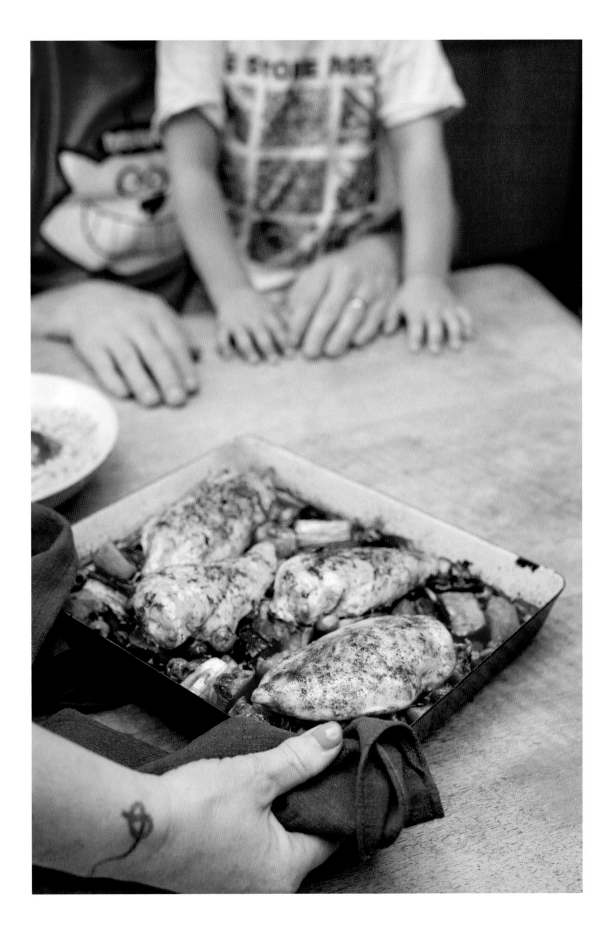

CHICKEN TAGINE TRAYBAKE

I've taken the flavourings from a classic North African tagine – saffron, spices, preserved lemons and olives – and used them in a low-effort chicken traybake. Just stick it in the oven and leave it to look after itself!

SERVES 4

400g sweet potatoes, peeled and cut into 4cm chunks
2 red onions, cut into wedges
2 garlic cloves, thinly sliced
2 preserved lemons, drained, roughly chopped and pips discarded
1 tbsp baharat seasoning
500ml fresh chicken stock
A large pinch of saffron strands, ground with a pestle and mortar
4 skinless boneless chicken breasts (180g each)
2 courgettes (320g), quartered lengthways and cut into 5cm pieces
100g pitted green olives
1-cal sunflower oil spray
Sea salt and freshly ground black pepper

For the couscous
150g couscous
200ml fresh chicken stock
A small pinch of saffron strands, ground with a pestle and mortar

Per serving: 532 cals
53g protein   57g carbs
9g fat   10g fibre

1 Preheat the oven to 220°C/Fan 200°C/Gas 7.

2 Put the sweet potatoes, onions, garlic and preserved lemons into a roasting tray. Sprinkle over half of the baharat, season liberally with salt and pepper, and mix well. Pour in half the stock and add the saffron. Cook on a high shelf in the oven for 25 minutes.

3 Rub some salt and the remaining baharat over both sides of the chicken breasts.

4 Take the roasting tray from the oven and add the courgettes, olives and remaining stock. Stir, then lay the chicken breasts on top and spray them with a few sprays of oil. Cook in the oven for 20–25 minutes until the chicken is cooked through.

5 Meanwhile, put the couscous into a small heatproof bowl and season with some salt and pepper. Heat the stock with the saffron then pour over the couscous. Cover and leave to stand for 15 minutes.

6 Fluff up the couscous gently with a fork and divide between bowls with the vegetables and chicken.

BONUS This is a really well-balanced meal to support your fitness, complete with protein, carbohydrates, vitamins and healthy fats from the olives. Sweet potatoes are also rich in beta-carotene, which helps muscles to recover after exercise.

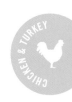

SAFFRON CHICKEN BURGERS

Burgers are the downfall of many dieters, so when those cravings strike, try this healthy version instead. Saffron gives the chicken an amazing colour and flavour, and it's a natural partner to harissa paste, which is a little hot and spicy.

SERVES 2

A pinch of saffron strands, ground with a pestle and mortar
1 tbsp boiling water
2 skinless boneless chicken breasts (180g each)
80g Greek yoghurt (0% fat)
2 garlic cloves, grated
1 tsp dried oregano
Sea salt and freshly ground black pepper

For the harissa yoghurt
100g Greek yoghurt (0% fat)
1 tsp harissa
A squeeze of lemon juice
A pinch of granulated sweetener

To assemble
2 wholemeal burger buns, lightly toasted
1 tomato, thickly sliced
6 thick slices cucumber
2 handfuls of mixed salad leaves

1 Preheat the oven to 230°C/Fan 220°C/Gas 8 with the grill element on. Line a baking tray with a silicone mat or baking paper.

2 Tip the saffron into a small heatproof bowl, pour on the boiling water and leave to stand.

3 Place each chicken breast between 2 sheets of cling film. Pound lightly with a rolling pin to a thickness of 1.5cm.

4 In a medium bowl, mix the yoghurt with the garlic, oregano and saffron water. Season with salt and pepper. Add the chicken breasts and turn to coat.

5 Place the chicken breasts on the lined tray and cook on a high shelf in the oven for 6 minutes, or until cooked through.

6 Meanwhile, for the harissa yoghurt, put the yoghurt into a bowl, add the harissa, lemon juice and sweetener and mix well, seasoning with a little salt and pepper.

7 Take the chicken from the oven and place on a metal tray. Run a cook's blowtorch over the surface of each breast to char lightly.

8 Spread each side of the burger buns with some harissa yoghurt. Place a chicken breast on each bun base, top with the tomato, cucumber and salad leaves and sandwich together with the bun tops.

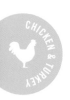
CHICKEN & TURKEY

Per serving: 420 cals
57g protein 32g carbs
6g fat 4g fibre

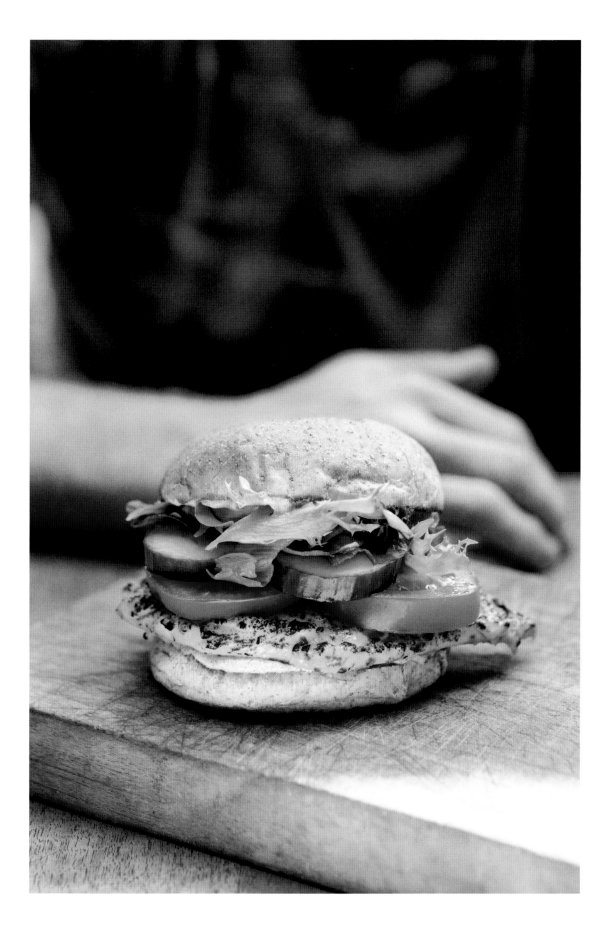

QUINOA TURKEY SCHNITZELS

 POST

Using quinoa instead of breadcrumbs to coat the turkey steaks for these schnitzels gives them a lovely crisp coating, as well as boosting the protein content.

SERVES 2

2 turkey steaks (170g each)
125g cooked quinoa (freshly cooked or ½ pouch), well drained
2 tsp garlic granules
1 tsp dried thyme
2 tbsp finely grated Parmesan (15g)
1 large free-range egg white (40g)
1-cal sunflower oil spray
Sea salt and freshly ground black pepper

For the garlic buttered veg

1 tbsp reduced-fat butter alternative
3 garlic cloves, finely chopped
200ml fresh chicken stock
200g tenderstem broccoli, trimmed
150g green beans, trimmed
80g frozen peas
Finely grated zest of ½ lemon

Per serving: *469 cals*
60g protein   *28g carbs*
11g fat   *12g fibre*

1 Preheat the oven to 230°C/Fan 220°C/Gas 8 with the grill element on.

2 Lay each turkey steak between 2 sheets of cling film. With a rolling pin, lightly pound each steak to an even 5mm thickness. Season all over with salt and pepper.

3 Put the cooked quinoa, garlic granules, thyme and grated Parmesan into a shallow bowl, along with some salt and pepper, and mix well.

4 In a separate shallow bowl, beat the egg white with a little seasoning, using a fork.

5 Dip each turkey steak into the egg white to coat both sides, then coat in the quinoa mixture, making sure both sides are fully covered.

6 Place a large ovenproof non-stick frying pan over a high heat and spray with oil. Add the turkey steaks and cook for 3–4 minutes, without turning – try not to move them. Spray the schnitzels with more oil, then place the pan on the highest oven shelf under the grill and cook for 4–5 minutes or until golden brown.

7 Meanwhile, prepare the garlic buttered veg. Melt the butter alternative in a sauté pan over a medium heat. Add the garlic and cook for 2 minutes. Pour in the stock, increase the heat and bring to a simmer. Add the broccoli and cook for 2 minutes. Add the beans and cook for a further 2 minutes. Add the peas and some salt and pepper and cook for a final 2 minutes. Take off the heat, add the lemon zest and serve alongside the turkey schnitzels.

CHICKEN & TURKEY

166

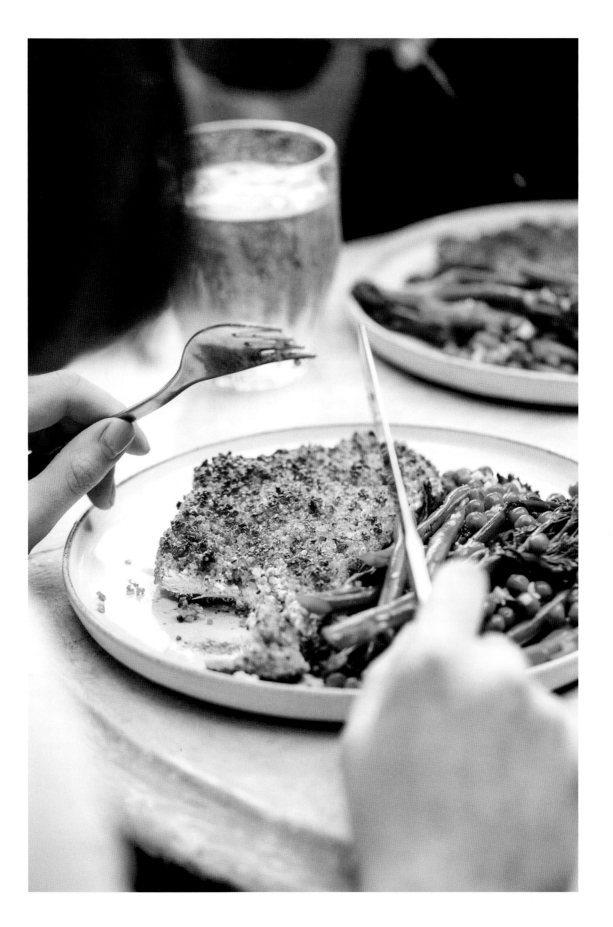

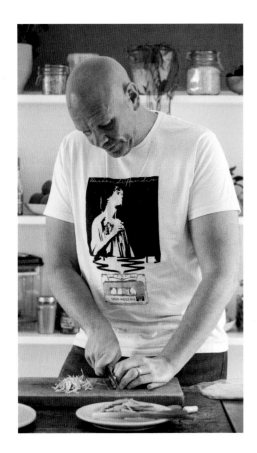

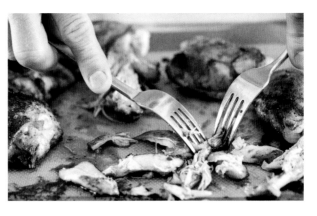

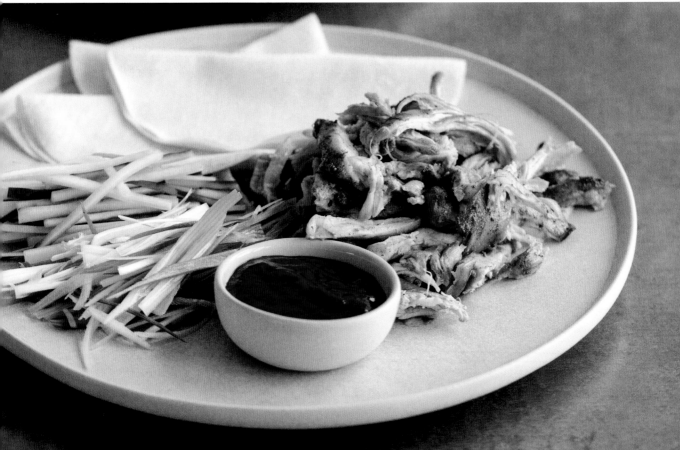

CHINESE-STYLE CHICKEN PANCAKES

This is a lower-calorie version of the classic Chinese dish that no one can resist; using chicken instead of duck lowers the fat content. Enjoy these pancakes at the weekend as a special treat.

SERVES 2

6 skinless chicken thighs
(bone in)
1 tsp Chinese five-spice
powder
1-cal sunflower oil spray
10–12 Chinese pancakes
Sea salt and freshly ground
white pepper

For the plum sauce
4 ripe plums (400g)
2 star anise
¼ tsp Sichuan peppercorns,
lightly crushed
1 garlic clove, grated
2cm piece fresh ginger, grated
1 tsp Chinese five-spice
powder
40ml red wine vinegar
1 tsp granulated sweetener
1 tsp soft brown sugar
50ml water
1 tbsp soy sauce

To serve
½ cucumber, julienned
3 spring onions, julienned

1 Preheat the oven to 200°C/Fan 180°C/Gas 6. Line a baking tray with a silicone mat or foil.

2 For the sauce, halve the plums, remove the stones then cut each half into 4 pieces. Place in a small pan with the star anise, Sichuan pepper, garlic, ginger, five-spice powder, wine vinegar, sweetener, sugar and water. Bring to the boil and simmer for 10 minutes or until the plums are softened and the liquid is reduced. Remove the star anise. Leave to cool slightly.

3 Tip the plum mixture into a small food processor and blend until smooth. Transfer to a bowl and season with the soy sauce and a little salt and pepper if needed.

4 To prepare the chicken thighs, rub them all over with the five-spice powder, season well with salt and white pepper and spray all over with oil. Place the chicken thighs on the lined tray and cook on a high shelf in the oven for 40–45 minutes or until browned and cooked through and the surface is a bit crispy.

5 Place the pancakes in a steamer over a pan of boiling water and warm through for a few minutes. Shred the chicken with 2 forks; discard the bones and any sinew.

6 Serve the pancakes, chicken, cucumber and spring onion on plates with the plum sauce. Assemble as you would duck pancakes at your local Chinese…

 BONUS For a lower-calorie option, use Little Gem lettuce leaves to wrap up your chicken in place of the pancakes. This will save you 166 calories.

Per serving: 676 cals
51g protein 53g carbs
28g fat 6g fibre

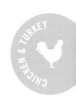

CHICKEN NOODLE SOUP

This chicken noodle soup is the first of three broths that use the same base to create different recipes. For a lighter meal and to boost your veg for the day, try it with spiralised courgettes and carrots instead of the egg noodles, as shown (see below). ❄

SERVES 4

1.5 litres fresh chicken stock
15g dried porcini mushrooms
1 star anise
2.5cm piece fresh ginger, thickly sliced
3 garlic cloves, lightly bashed
3 spring onions, white and green parts separated
750g skinless chicken thighs (bone in)

To assemble

100ml shaoxing wine
2 tbsp soy sauce
1 tbsp oyster sauce
180g fine egg noodles
200g choi sum, cut into 7.5cm lengths
Sea salt and freshly ground white pepper

To serve

80g bamboo shoots
1 tsp sesame oil

Per serving: *450 cals*
39g protein   *37g carbs*
15g fat   *6g fibre*

1 Pour the stock into a medium saucepan, place over a high heat and add the dried porcini, star anise, ginger, garlic and white spring onions. Add the chicken thighs to the pan, bring to a gentle simmer and cook gently for 25 minutes or until the chicken is tender.

2 Pour the broth through a strainer into a jug, remove the chicken from the strainer and set aside; discard the rest of the contents. Return the broth to the pan and bring back to the boil over a medium-high heat. Allow to reduce for 5 minutes to intensify the flavour.

3 Meanwhile, shred the chicken meat, discarding the bones. Finely shred the green parts of the spring onions and set aside for the garnish.

4 Stir the shaoxing wine, soy and oyster sauces into the broth. Season with a little salt if needed, and white pepper to taste. Add the egg noodles and cook until tender. Lift out the noodles and divide them between warmed bowls.

5 Add the chicken and choi sum to the pan, cook for 2 minutes to warm through and wilt the choi sum then lift out and add to the bowls with the bamboo shoots and green spring onions. Ladle in the broth and drizzle with a little sesame oil to serve.

TO FREEZE Follow the directions for the broth overleaf.

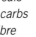 **BONUS** Replacing the egg noodles with 200g each of spiralised carrot and courgette saves you 130 calories.

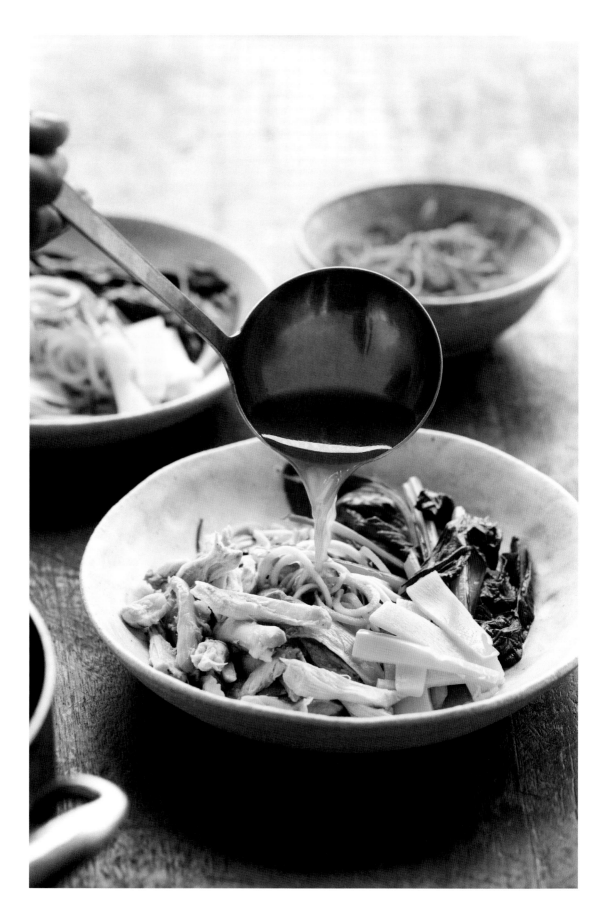

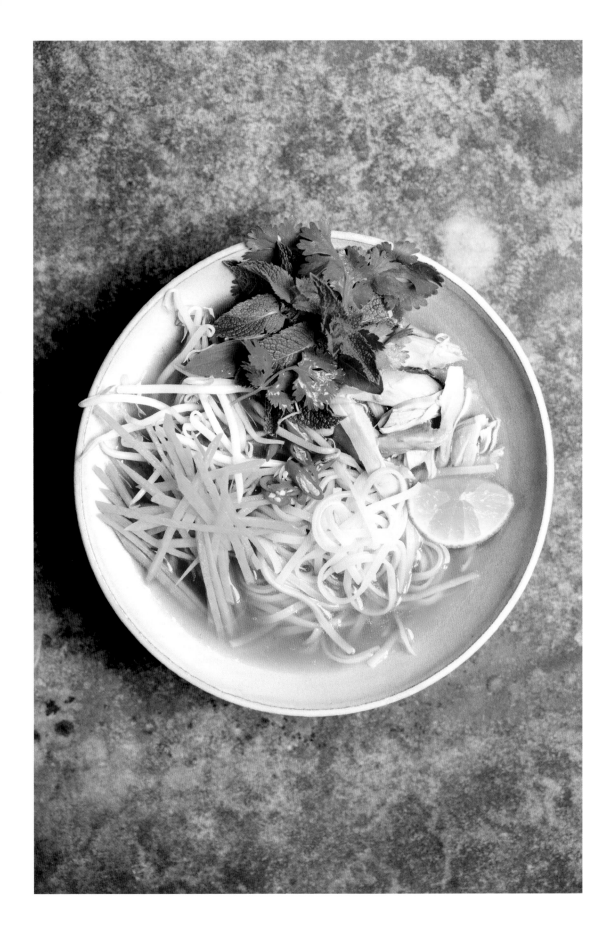

CHICKEN PHO

This Vietnamese pho is full of aromatic flavours, such as cinnamon, coriander, ginger and lemongrass, and topped with loads of fresh herbs. Feel free to play about with the seasoning and spices to find the perfect balance for you. ❄

SERVES 4

1.5 litres fresh chicken stock
15g dried porcini mushrooms
2.5cm piece fresh ginger, thickly sliced
3 garlic cloves, lightly bashed
1 star anise
¼ tsp black peppercorns
¼ tsp Chinese five-spice powder
1 tsp coriander seeds
1 cinnamon stick
2 lemongrass stems, lightly bashed
3 spring onions, white and green parts separated
750g skinless chicken thighs (bone in)
200g carrots, julienned
200g flat rice noodles
2 tbsp fish sauce
Juice of 1 lime
Sea salt and freshly ground white pepper

To finish and serve

200g beansprouts
A large handful each of mint, coriander and Thai basil
1 bird's eye chilli, finely sliced
1 lime, cut into wedges

Per serving: *485 cals*
39g protein   *48g carbs*
14g fat   *6g fibre*

1 Pour the stock into a medium saucepan, place over a high heat and add the dried porcini, ginger, garlic, spices, lemongrass and white spring onions. Add the chicken thighs, bring to a low simmer and cook gently for 25 minutes or until the chicken is tender.

2 Meanwhile, put the carrot julienne and rice noodles into a large heatproof bowl, pour on boiling water to cover generously and leave to soften for 10 minutes. Finely shred the green spring onions for the garnish.

3 Pour the broth through a strainer into a jug, remove the chicken from the strainer and set aside for later; discard the rest of the contents. Return the flavoured broth to the pan and place over a medium-high heat.

4 Bring back to the boil and let bubble for 5 minutes to reduce and intensify the flavour. Stir in the fish sauce and lime juice. Season the soup with a pinch of sea salt if needed and a small pinch of white pepper.

5 Shred the chicken, discarding the bones, then add to the broth to warm through for 2 minutes. Drain the noodles and carrot and share between warmed bowls. Scoop the chicken out of the pan and add to the bowls. Ladle over the broth and finish with the spring onions, beansprouts, herbs, chilli and lime wedges.

TO FREEZE Allow the strained broth to cool at the end of stage 4 then freeze in a suitable container. Shred the chicken and freeze separately. Defrost both at room temperature, then reheat the broth thoroughly in a pan over a medium heat. Continue as above.

173

CHICKEN, MISO AND MUSHROOM RAMEN

A popular Japanese dish, ramen is an intensely flavoured noodle broth topped with meat or vegetables. This chicken version is flavoured with soy, miso and mushrooms and finished with a boiled egg. Go ahead and add as much fresh chilli as you like! ❄

SERVES 4

1.5 litres fresh chicken stock
15g dried porcini mushrooms
1 star anise
2.5cm piece fresh ginger, thickly sliced
3 garlic cloves, lightly bashed
3 spring onions, white and green parts separated
750g skinless chicken thighs (bone in)
4 large free-range eggs
2 tbsp white miso paste
1 tbsp mirin
1 tbsp soy sauce
12 dried shiitake mushrooms
400g cooked ramen noodles
100g baby spinach
Sea salt and freshly ground white pepper

To finish

1 red chilli, deseeded and cut into thin strips
1 tsp furikake (Japanese seasoning)

Per serving: 535 cals
49g protein   37g carbs
20g fat   5g fibre

1 Pour the stock into a medium saucepan, place over a high heat and add the dried porcini, star anise, ginger, garlic and white parts of the spring onions. Add the chicken thighs to the pan, bring the stock to a gentle simmer and cook gently for 25 minutes or until the chicken is tender.

2 Pour the broth through a strainer into a jug, remove the chicken from the strainer and set aside for later; discard the rest of the contents. Return the flavoured broth to the pan and place over a medium-high heat.

3 When the broth comes to the boil, carefully add the eggs (in their shells) and cook for 6 minutes. Lift them out and place in a bowl of cold water to cool slightly.

4 Whisk the miso paste into the broth, then stir in the mirin and soy. Add the dried shiitake mushrooms and cook for 3–4 minutes or until they are tender. Meanwhile, finely shred the green parts of the spring onions for the garnish. Season the soup with a pinch of sea salt and a small pinch of white pepper.

5 Add the cooked ramen noodles to the broth and warm through, then lift out and divide between 4 warmed bowls. Shred the chicken, discarding any bones, then add it to the broth to warm through. Scoop out the chicken and add to the bowls. Drop the spinach into the broth and let it wilt, then lift out and add to the bowls as well.

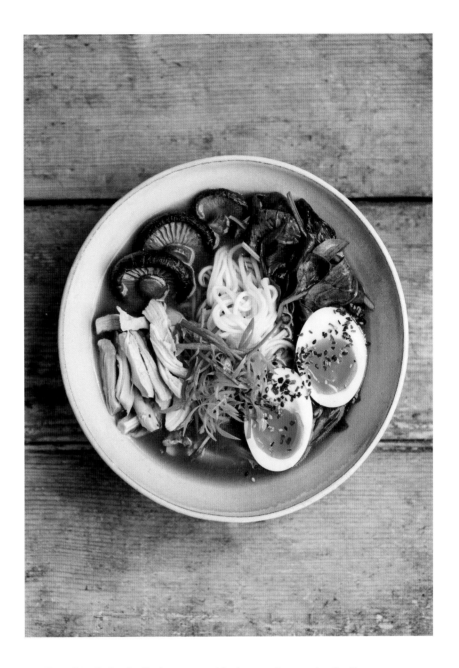

6 Shell the boiled eggs and halve each one. Ladle the broth into the bowls, add the eggs, and garnish with the spring onions, red chilli and furikake.

TO FREEZE Let the strained broth cool at the end of stage 4 then freeze in a suitable container. Shred the chicken and freeze separately. Defrost both at room temperature, then reheat the broth thoroughly in a pan over a medium heat. Continue as for the recipe.

CHICKEN AND YOGHURT CURRY

 POST Ideal for a hearty midweek supper, this easy curry is packed with clean, uncomplicated flavours and it's quick to make. ❄

SERVES 4

2 tsp olive oil
1 onion, finely chopped
A small bunch of coriander, stalks and leaves separated
6 garlic cloves, finely chopped
5cm piece fresh ginger, finely grated
1 long green chilli, finely chopped (with seeds)
2 tsp ground cumin
2 tsp ground coriander
1 tsp ground turmeric
2 tbsp tomato purée
500ml fresh chicken stock
1kg skinless boneless chicken thighs, cut into 5cm pieces
200g full-fat Greek yoghurt
150g baby spinach
Sea salt and freshly ground black pepper
500g cooked brown basmati rice (freshly cooked and drained or 2 pouches), to serve

1 Heat the oil in a large non-stick sauté pan over a high heat. Add the onion and cook for 5–7 minutes or until golden brown. Meanwhile, finely chop the coriander stalks; set the leaves aside for later.

2 Add the garlic, ginger and chilli to the pan and cook for 2 minutes. Sprinkle in the spices with 1 tsp salt and cook, stirring, for 1 minute. Stir in the tomato purée and cook, stirring, for 2 minutes. Toss in the chopped coriander stalks and cook for 1 minute.

3 Pour in the stock, bring to a simmer and let simmer for 5 minutes before adding the chicken pieces to the pan. Stir well and cook gently for 25 minutes, or until the sauce is thickened and the chicken is tender and cooked through. (Aim for a thicker than usual curry consistency, as you will be adding yoghurt.)

4 Meanwhile, if using pouches of rice, heat up according to the packet instructions and chop the coriander leaves. Stir the yoghurt and spinach through the curry and cook for 2–3 minutes until the spinach is wilted.

5 Season the curry with salt and pepper to taste and add the coriander. Serve in warmed bowls, with the rice.

TO FREEZE Allow to cool then freeze in portions. Defrost fully overnight in the fridge, then reheat gently in a pan over a medium heat until hot all the way through.

 BONUS Served with rice, this curry ticks off all the food groups. It is an ideal mix of protein and carbs along with iron, vitamins and minerals – just what you need for a speedy post-workout recovery.

Per serving: *708 cals*
59g protein   *45g carbs*
32g fat   *4g fibre*

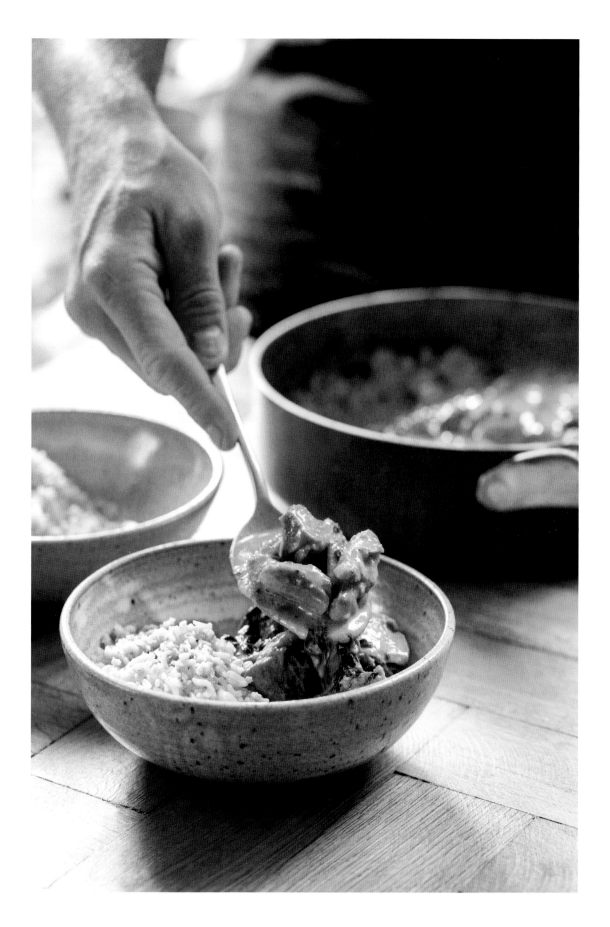

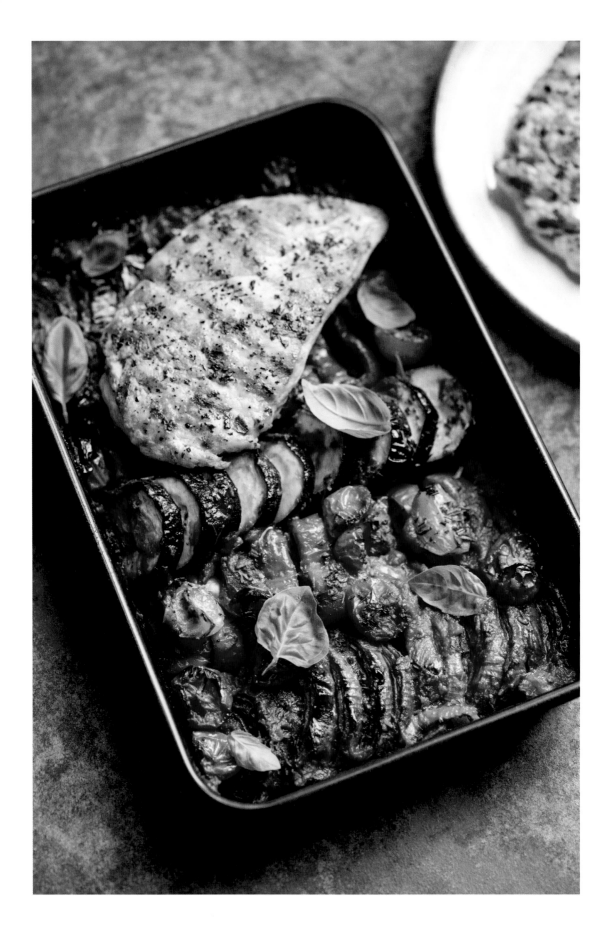

CHICKEN RATATOUILLE

Ratatouille brings together lovely Mediterranean flavours that go well with chicken. The trick here is to layer in as much texture as possible, keeping the veg quite chunky so each one can sing.

SERVES 2

2 Romano peppers, halved, cored and deseeded
1 courgette (200g)
1 red onion (120g), halved
½ aubergine (150g), halved lengthways
200g passata
1 garlic clove, grated
½ tsp Italian seasoning
1 tbsp extra-virgin olive oil
200g cherry tomatoes, halved (mixed colours)
2 sprigs of rosemary, leaves stripped and finely chopped
2 skinless boneless chicken breasts (180g each)
2 sprigs of oregano, leaves stripped and finely chopped
1-cal olive oil spray
Sea salt and freshly ground black pepper
Basil leaves, to garnish

1 Preheat the oven to 230°C/Fan 220°C/Gas 8. Slice the peppers into 1cm-thick rings, the courgette into 1cm-thick rounds and the red onion and aubergine into 1cm-thick half-moons.

2 In a bowl, mix the passata with the garlic, Italian seasoning and a little salt and pepper. Spread over the base of a 20 x 25cm oven dish.

3 Lay the veg in lines across the dish, overlapping the slices. Brush the surface with the extra-virgin olive oil and season well with salt and pepper, then scatter the cherry tomatoes and rosemary over the top. Cook in the oven for 20–25 minutes.

4 Place each chicken breast between 2 sheets of cling film. Using a rolling pin, lightly pound the thicker areas so the chicken breasts are an even thickness (about 2cm). Sprinkle both sides with oregano, salt and pepper.

5 Place a non-stick griddle pan over a medium-high heat. When it is hot, spray the chicken breasts a few times with olive oil and lay on the griddle. Cook for 3–4 minutes on each side or until golden brown and cooked through, pressing them down as they cook so they get good char marks.

6 Serve the chicken with the roasted ratatouille, scattered with basil leaves.

Per serving: *383 cals*
46g protein *20g carbs*
11g fat *10g fibre*

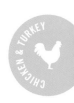

CHICKEN & TURKEY

TURKEY MEATBALLS IN ROASTED PEPPER SAUCE

Turkey mince is a lower-fat alternative to beef in these tasty meatballs. It also takes on other flavours really well, like the sweet roasted peppers in the sauce. ❄

 POST

SERVES 4

500g turkey mince
2 garlic cloves, grated
2 tsp dried oregano
1 large free-range egg,
  lightly beaten
1-cal olive oil spray

For the sauce
2 tsp olive oil
1 onion, finely chopped
2 garlic cloves, sliced
3 tbsp tomato purée
1 tsp sweet smoked paprika
1 tsp paprika
400g whole roasted peppers
  (from a jar), roughly
  chopped
400ml fresh chicken stock
2 courgettes, diced
50ml single cream
A small handful of basil leaves,
  roughly chopped
Sea salt and freshly ground
  black pepper

To serve
500g cooked wholegrain or
  five-grain rice (freshly
  cooked and drained or
  2 pouches)

Per serving: 531 cals
47g protein   45g carbs
17g fat   4g fibre

1 Preheat the oven to 230°C/Fan 220°C/Gas 8 with the grill element on. Line a baking tray with a silicone mat or baking paper.

2 Put the turkey mince, garlic, dried oregano and egg into a large bowl and season generously with salt and pepper. Mix together with your hands. Take a small nugget of the mixture and cook it in a small frying pan then taste for seasoning and adjust the mixture accordingly.

3 Divide the mixture into 20 even-sized pieces and roll into balls. Spread the meatballs out on the lined tray and cook on a high shelf in the oven for 5 minutes. (You're not really looking to get any colour on them at this stage, it just helps them hold together.)

4 In the meantime, for the sauce, place a large sauté pan over a high heat and add the oil. When hot, add the onion and cook for 4 minutes or until softened. Add the garlic and cook for 2–3 minutes. Stir in the tomato purée and both paprikas and cook, stirring, for 2 minutes. Add the roasted peppers, pour in the stock and simmer for 5 minutes.

5 Transfer the sauce to a jug blender and blend until smooth. Season with salt and pepper to taste.

6 Add the sauce to the sauté pan and bring to a gentle simmer. Add the courgettes and cook for 2 minutes, then stir in the cream and basil. Add the meatballs to the sauce and simmer for a few minutes to reheat; check that they are cooked right through.

CHICKEN & TURKEY

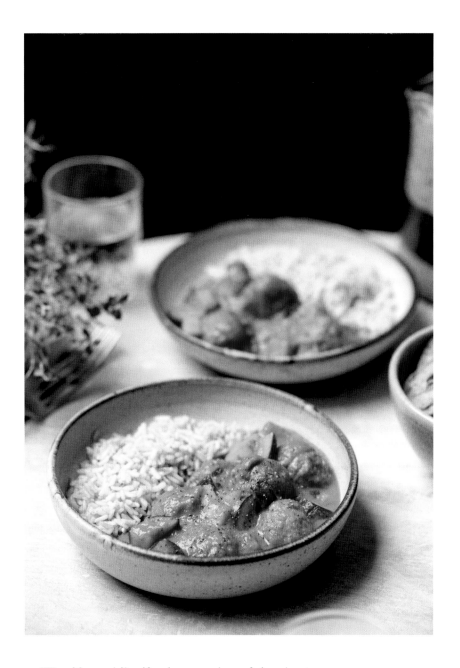

7 Meanwhile, if using pouches of rice, heat up according to the packet instructions. Serve the meatballs and sauce with the wholegrain rice.

TO FREEZE Allow to cool, then freeze in two-portion foil trays with foil lids. Defrost fully in the fridge overnight. Reheat, covered, in an oven preheated to 200°C/ Fan 180°C/Gas 6 for 30 minutes or until piping hot.

CHICKEN, BROWN RICE AND LENTIL PILAF

I know this pilaf sounds like it might be the healthiest thing on earth and you don't always associate healthy dishes with loads of flavour, but the spicing that goes into this makes it exciting. It is wholesome and satisfying but won't leave you feeling stuffed.

SERVES 2

1 tsp vegetable oil
1 onion, finely diced
2 garlic cloves, finely chopped
1.5cm piece fresh ginger, finely grated
250g skinless boneless chicken thighs, cut into 1–2cm dice
½ tsp ground cumin
½ tsp ground coriander
1 tsp garam masala
200ml fresh chicken stock
150g tenderstem broccoli, roughly chopped
100g frozen peas
150g cooked Puy lentils (freshly cooked or from a pouch)
250g cooked brown and wild rice (freshly cooked and drained or a pouch)
50g baby spinach
A handful of coriander leaves, chopped
Sea salt and freshly ground black pepper

1 Heat the oil in a medium non-stick sauté pan over a medium heat. When hot, add the onion and cook for 4–5 minutes or until softened and starting to brown. Add the garlic and ginger and cook for 2 minutes.

2 Add the diced chicken to the sauté pan and cook for 3–4 minutes, stirring regularly. Add a splash of stock if it starts to stick. Stir in the spices and cook, stirring, for 1 minute. Pour in the stock, bring to a simmer and cook for 5 minutes.

3 Add the broccoli to the pan and cook for 2 minutes, then add the peas, cooked lentils and cooked rice. Stir well, put the lid on the sauté pan and cook for 3–4 minutes to steam the broccoli.

4 Stir through the spinach and chopped coriander, season well with salt and pepper and cook until the spinach is just wilted. Serve in warmed bowls.

BONUS Chicken and lentils provide two different protein sources, making this a top choice for helping your muscles recover after a heavy workout. Puy lentils are also a good source of iron and fibre.

Per serving: *691 cals*
49g protein   *72g carbs*
19g fat   *17g fibre*

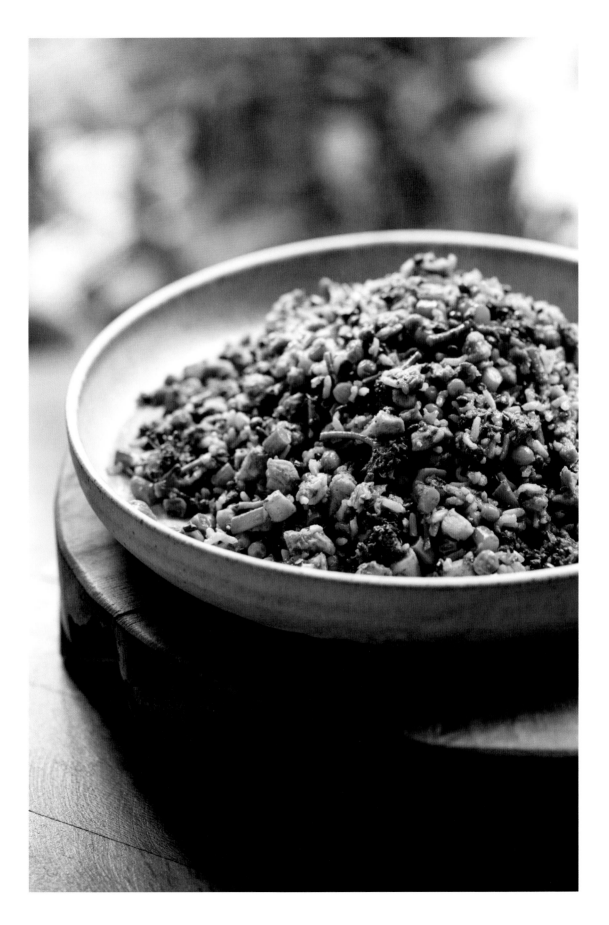

PAPRIKA CHICKEN

Paprika is my go-to seasoning of choice after salt and pepper.
I love the smokiness you get from it and the rich dark colour
it brings to dishes. This simple and quick, full-flavoured recipe
uses mostly store-cupboard ingredients so it's a great choice for
a midweek meal.

SERVES 2

2 skinless boneless chicken
    breasts (180g each)
2 tsp olive oil
2 banana shallots, finely
    chopped
2 garlic cloves, finely sliced
1 tsp sweet smoked paprika
2 tsp paprika
1 tbsp tomato purée
50ml dry sherry
250ml fresh chicken stock
300g green vegetables (such
    as tenderstem broccoli,
    green beans and peas)
2 tbsp full-fat crème fraîche
1 tbsp finely chopped flat-leaf
    parsley
Sea salt and freshly ground
    black pepper

1 Place each chicken breast between 2 sheets of cling
film. Using a rolling pin, lightly pound the thicker
areas so the chicken breasts are an even thickness
(about 2cm). Season all over with salt and pepper.

2 Heat half the oil in a large non-stick frying pan over
a high heat. Add the chicken breasts and cook for
2 minutes on each side. Remove the chicken from
the pan and transfer to a plate.

3 Add the remaining olive oil to the frying pan over
a medium-high heat. Add the shallots and cook for
2–3 minutes or until softened, stirring regularly.
Toss in the garlic and cook for 2 minutes. Stir in both
paprikas and cook for 30 seconds then stir in the
tomato purée and cook, stirring, for 1 minute.

4 Add the sherry and let it bubble to reduce right down
before pouring in the stock. Bring to a simmer and
allow to bubble until the liquor is reduced by half.

5 Meanwhile, place a steamer over a pan of boiling
water. Add the vegetables and steam for 5 minutes
or until tender.

6 Add the chicken to the sauce and simmer gently for
2–3 minutes until cooked through. Stir in the crème
fraîche and season with salt and pepper to taste. Stir
through the chopped parsley and serve with the
steamed vegetables alongside.

Per serving: *399 cals*
50g protein   *7g carbs*
14g fat   *7g fibre*

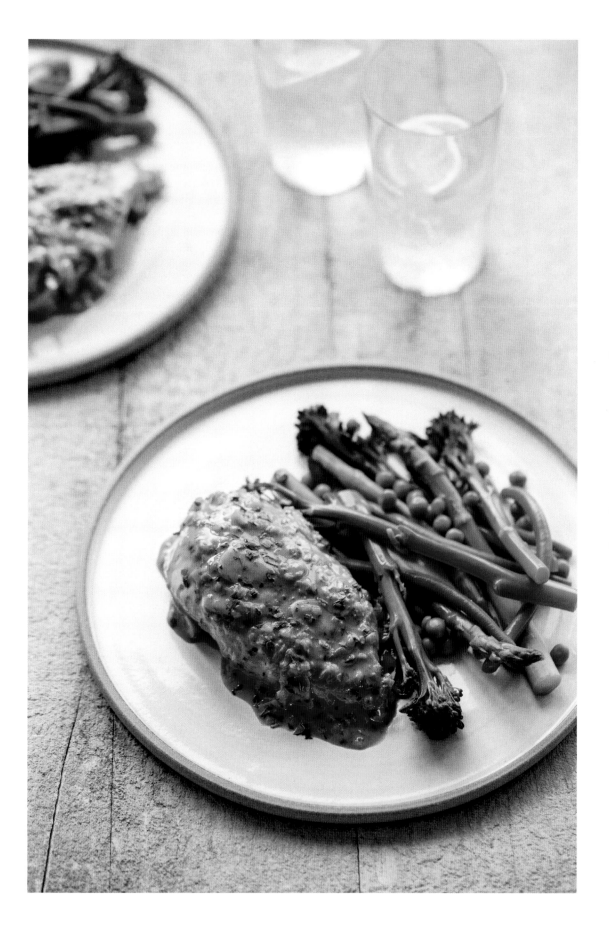

TURKEY SAUSAGES AND BEANS

Making your own sausages takes a bit of work, but these are a great, lighter alternative to the usual pork version. Don't worry about getting them all perfectly even, it's all about the flavour with this recipe.

SERVES 4

For the sausages
1 tsp olive oil
1 onion, finely chopped
3 garlic cloves, finely chopped
½ tsp fennel seeds
½ tsp dried chilli flakes
1 tbsp finely chopped sage
500g turkey thigh mince
1 large free-range egg
1 tsp sea salt
½ tsp coarsely ground black
    pepper
1-cal sunflower oil spray

For the beans in tomato sauce
1 tsp olive oil
2 shallots, finely diced
2 tbsp finely chopped rosemary
1 tsp paprika
1 tbsp tomato purée
500ml fresh chicken stock
200g whole roasted red
    peppers (from a jar), diced
250g cherry tomatoes, halved
3 x 400g tins cannellini beans,
    drained and rinsed
100g baby spinach
Sea salt and freshly ground
    black pepper

Per serving: *498 cals*
57g protein   *31g carbs*
13g fat   *15g fibre*

1 To make the sausages, heat the olive oil in a small non-stick frying pan over a medium heat. When hot, add the onion and cook for 3–4 minutes until softened. Add the garlic and cook for 2 minutes, then stir in the fennel seeds, chilli flakes and chopped sage. Cook, stirring, for 1 minute then remove from the heat and leave to cool slightly.

2 Put the turkey mince and egg into a food processor with the salt and pepper. Blend to a smooth paste then add the cooled onion mix and pulse a few times to combine. Take a small nugget of the mixture and cook it in a small frying pan, then taste to check the seasoning and adjust the mixture accordingly.

3 Cut 8 pieces of cling film, each about 35 x 20cm. Take the mixture from the food processor and divide it into 8 even-sized pieces. Wet your hands (to stop the mixture sticking to them) then roll each piece into a sausage and wrap tightly in a piece of cling film, twisting the ends and tying them in knots to seal.

4 Bring a large pan of water to the boil. Add the cling-film-wrapped sausages and lay a round of baking paper over the surface – to ensure they remain submerged in the water and cook through properly. Bring the water back to a simmer and poach the sausages for 8 minutes.

Continued overleaf

186

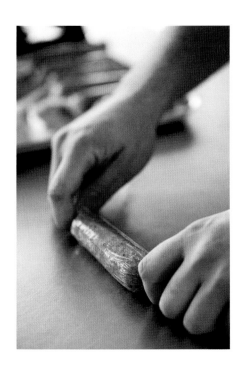

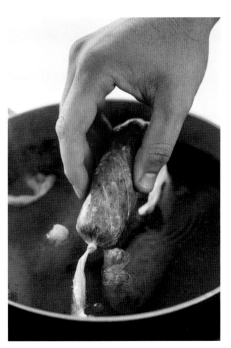

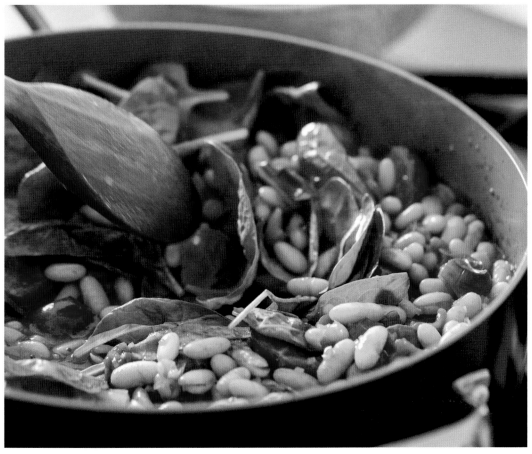

5 Meanwhile, prepare the beans. Heat the olive oil in a large sauté pan over a medium heat then add the shallots and cook for 4–5 minutes or until softened. Add the rosemary and cook for another minute.

6 Add the paprika and tomato purée to the shallots, stir and cook for 2 minutes then pour in the stock. Bring to a simmer and simmer steadily for 10 minutes or until the liquor is reduced by half. Add the red peppers, tomatoes and beans to the pan along with some seasoning and cook for 15 minutes or until the sauce has thickened slightly.

7 In the meantime, lift the sausages out of the water onto a board and leave them to rest for a few minutes. When they are cool enough to handle, unwrap the sausages, discarding the cling film. Place a large non-stick frying pan over a high heat and add a few sprays of oil. Place the sausages in the pan and fry for 4–5 minutes or until golden brown all over.

8 Add the spinach to the beans, stir well and cook for 2–3 minutes or until the spinach is wilted. Season with salt and pepper to taste.

9 Divide the beans between warmed shallow bowls and top each serving with a couple of sausages.

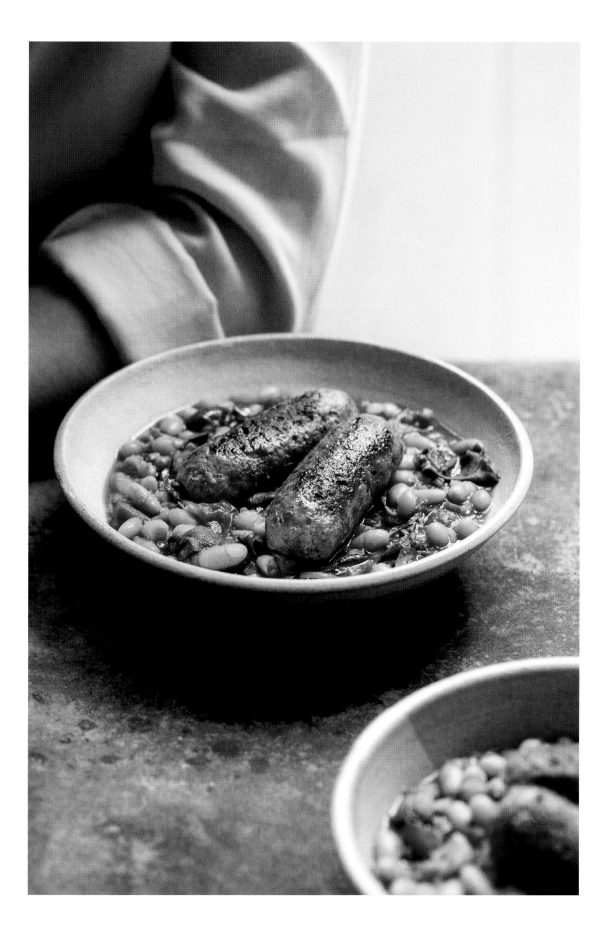

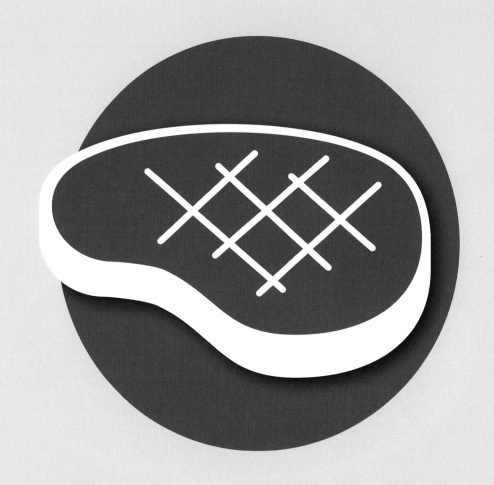

7 BEEF, LAMB & PORK

WE ALL KNOW MEAT IS TASTY and satisfying, but it's often quite high in fat and calories. However, it is a great source of protein and other nutrients that can help you reach your fitness goals, and it can really make you feel like you've eaten a substantial meal too – which I know is half the battle when you're on a diet. When you're cutting back on calories, the trick is to try and make meat go a bit further in your cooking, using leaner cuts where you can – such as lean mince and stewing steak – and by focusing on the other flavours and textures in the dish as well.

It helps to see meat as a bit more of a treat, rather than something you eat every day, and to serve it alongside lots of tasty veg. So don't worry: your favourite steak supper is definitely still very much in play! In fact, steak – trimmed of any fat – is great for quick cooking. It's brilliant in stir-fries, such as my black pepper stir-fry on page 192, and you won't need to use very much of it either, as there's so much else going on with all the veg and intense flavours in the sauce. I've also used lean steak in the tacos with corn salsa on page 194, which are perfect for sharing if you have people round.

The smoky beef chilli on page 197 serves up a really generously sized portion, but it's relatively lower in calories because it's jam-packed full of beans and veg. The chilli actually uses the same basic mince mixture that I use in the cottage pie and beef ragu with pasta on pages 202 and 208. These are three of the most popular dishes you'll find in many people's cooking repertoire, so I wanted to show you how to take a simple beef ragu and flavour it up three ways to create delicious, healthy versions of these regular standbys. Roasting the mince first is a clever way to add an extra layer of flavour without adding calories – it takes a little bit longer, but it's really worth it. You could even make a big batch of the mince mixture and freeze it, so you'll already be halfway towards a comforting midweek meal.

If you're worried about missing out on your traditional Sunday roast, then the pork loin with celeriac, garlic and cider on page 214 is a healthy alternative – OK, so there are no Yorkies to be found here, but the juices from the pan and the deliciously tender meat will more than make up for it.

You really don't need to miss out on meat when you're losing weight; it's completely possible to make meat a healthy part of your new way of eating with a few easy adjustments.

BLACK PEPPER BEEF STIR-FRY

Stir-fries are a brilliant option when you need healthy food fast. You just need to get everything prepped and ready to go before you start cooking. The cornflour gives the fiery black pepper sauce body without adding lots of extra calories.

SERVES 2

300g rump steak, trimmed of any fat
1 tsp vegetable oil
1 red onion, finely sliced
2 garlic cloves, finely sliced
5cm piece fresh ginger, julienned
1 red pepper, cored, deseeded and thinly sliced
1 green pepper, cored, deseeded and thinly sliced
1 tsp cornflour
2 tbsp oyster sauce
1 tbsp soy sauce
2 tbsp shaoxing wine

For the marinade
1 tsp cornflour
1 tsp soy sauce
1 tsp sesame oil
A good pinch of flaky sea salt
½ tsp coarsely ground black pepper

To serve
250g cooked brown rice (freshly cooked and drained or a pouch)
2 spring onions, green part only, finely shredded

Per serving: 526 cals
41g protein   58g carbs
13g fat   7g fibre

1 Slice the steak thinly, into 5mm thick slices. For the marinade, combine all the ingredients in a bowl. Add the steak slices, toss to mix and leave to marinate for a few minutes.

2 Place a wok over a high heat. When it starts to smoke, add half the oil followed by half of the beef. Stir-fry very quickly for 1–2 minutes, then remove the beef from the pan to a plate. Add the rest of the oil to the wok and repeat with the remaining meat.

3 Put the wok back over a high heat. Add the onion and cook for 2 minutes, then add the garlic and ginger and stir-fry for 1 minute, adding a little water to prevent sticking if needed. Add the peppers and stir-fry for a further 2–3 minutes.

4 Meanwhile, if using a pouch of rice, heat up according to the packet instructions. Mix the cornflour to a paste with 2 tbsp water.

5 Add the oyster and soy sauces, shaoxing wine and ½ tsp black pepper to the wok and stir to combine. Return the beef to the wok, along with any resting juices. Now stir in the cornflour paste and stir-fry for another minute or until the sauce is thickened and the beef is warmed through.

6 Divide the rice between warmed bowls and top with the stir-fry. Finish with a scattering of shredded green spring onion.

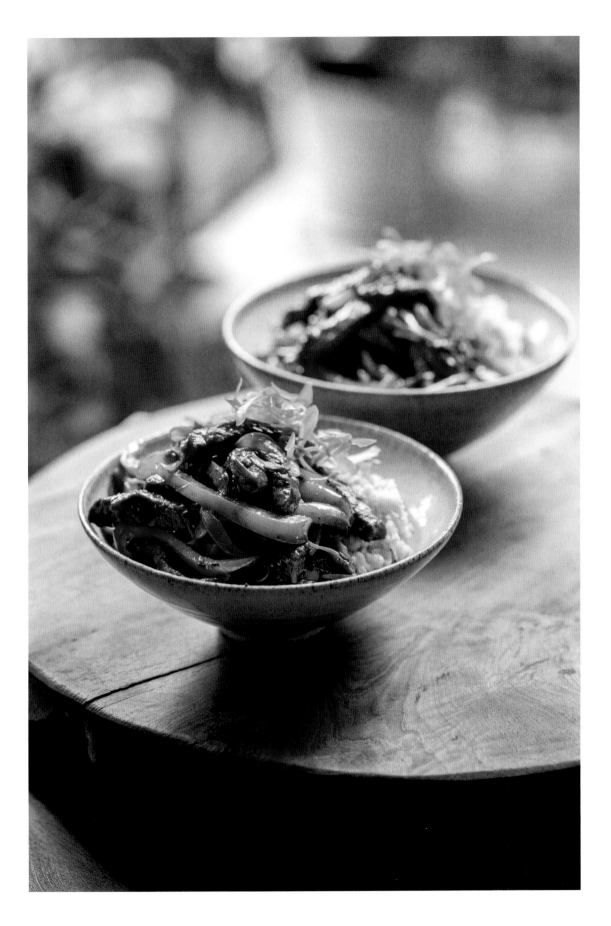

STEAK TACOS WITH BURNT CORN SALSA

Bavette steak is economical, and a little goes a long way in these hugely flavoursome tacos. The colourful roasted corn salsa and tacos are finished with a cooling avocado cream – there are so many exciting tastes and textures working together here. Enjoy!

SERVES 2

2 bavette steaks (150g each)
1 tsp ground cumin
½ tsp chilli powder
½ tsp dried oregano
1-cal sunflower oil spray
Sea salt and freshly ground
    black pepper

For the burnt corn salsa
1 corn-on-the-cob
1-cal sunflower oil spray
½ red onion, finely diced
1 fresh green jalapeño pepper,
    finely diced
8 cherry tomatoes, quartered
A small handful of coriander,
    roughly chopped (including
    stalks)
Juice of ½ lime

For the avocado crema
½ ripe avocado
50ml reduced-fat soured
    cream
Juice of ½ lime, or to taste

To assemble
4 Mexican corn (or blue corn)
    tortillas, 15cm in diameter

Per serving: 600 cals
38g protein   39g carbs
31g fat   6g fibre

1 Lay the steaks on a board. Mix the cumin, chilli powder and oregano together with 1 tsp salt. Sprinkle evenly over both sides of the steaks. Set aside.

2 To prepare the burnt corn salsa, stand the corn cob upright on a board and run a sharp knife down the sides to release the kernels.

3 Add a few sprays of oil to a medium non-stick frying pan and place over a high heat. When hot, add the corn kernels and cook for 4 minutes or until starting to brown. Add the red onion and jalapeño pepper, cook for 2 minutes then take off the heat. Tip into a bowl and add the cherry tomatoes, coriander and lime juice. Season with salt and pepper to taste.

4 For the avocado crema, in a small bowl, mash the avocado with the soured cream. Season with salt and pepper and stir in the lime juice to taste.

5 Heat a large non-stick frying pan over a high heat, then add a few sprays of oil followed by the steaks. Cook for 3–4 minutes on each side. Remove from the pan and leave to rest in a warm spot.

6 Place 2 large non-stick frying pans over a high heat. When hot, add a tortilla to each pan and heat for 30 seconds or so on each side. Remove and repeat with the remaining tortillas.

7 Slice the steaks thickly and serve on the warmed tortillas, along with the salsa and avocado crema.

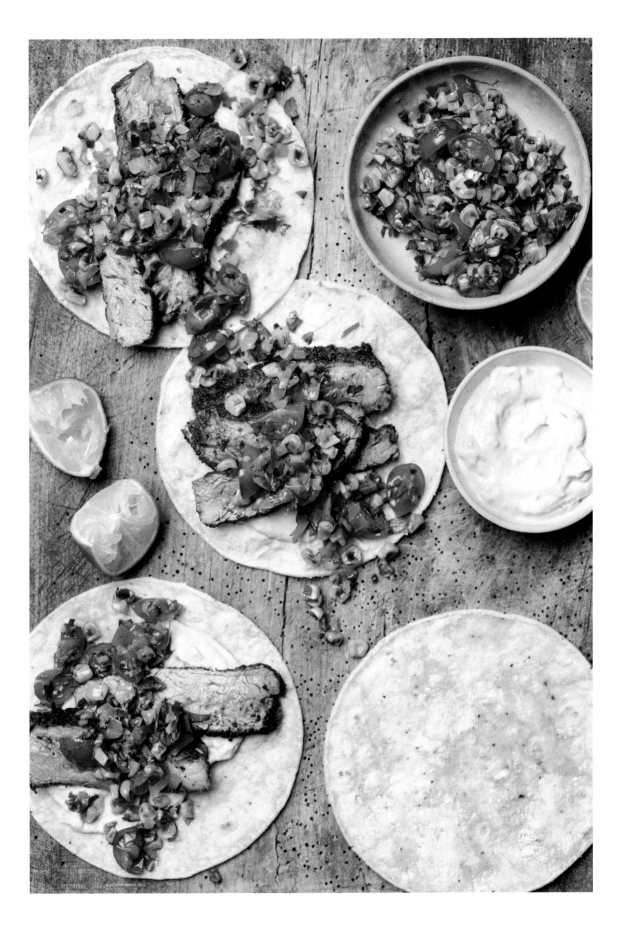

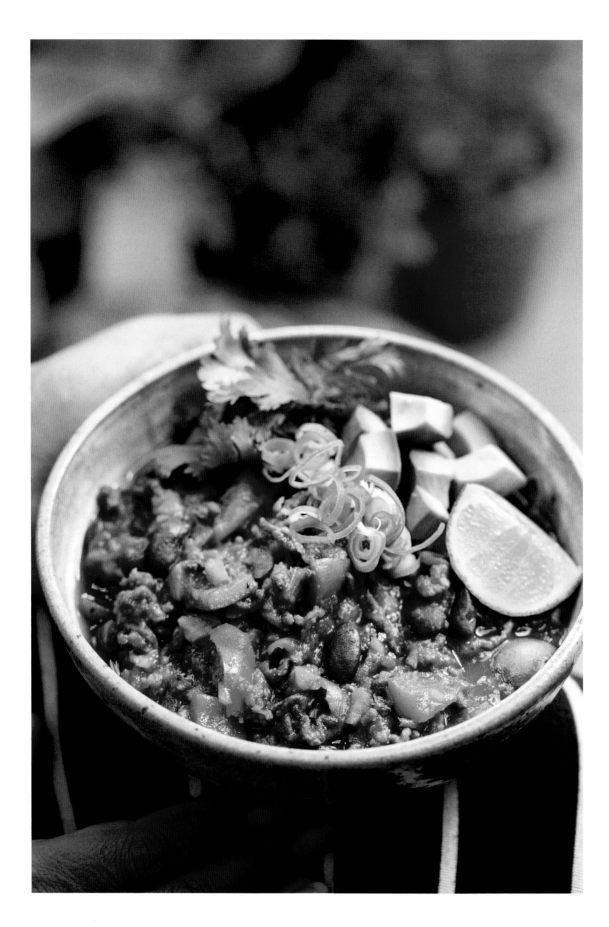

SMOKY BEEF CHILLI

Most chilli recipes include dried chilli powder and although they might taste great, I can guarantee this one will taste even better because it uses hot and smoky chipotle paste instead. ✳

SERVES 8

1kg lean beef mince (5% fat)
2 large onions, quartered
250g carrots, cut into chunks
150g celery sticks, cut into
   short lengths
6 garlic cloves, halved
1 tbsp vegetable oil
1 tbsp ground cumin
1 tsp hot smoked paprika
½ tsp ground cinnamon
2 tbsp chipotle paste
1 litre fresh beef stock
1 tsp dried oregano
2 x 400g tins kidney beans,
   drained and rinsed (480g
   total drained weight)
2 x 400g tins chopped
   tomatoes
1 red pepper, cored, deseeded
   and diced
1 green pepper, cored,
   deseeded and diced

To finish
1 ripe avocado, diced
4 spring onions, finely sliced
A large handful of coriander
   leaves
1 lime, cut into wedges

Per serving: *395 cals*
46g protein   *21g carbs*
12g fat   *10g fibre*

1 Preheat the oven to 200°C/Fan 180°C/Gas 6. Line a baking tray with a silicone mat or baking paper.

2 Spread the beef mince out evenly on the lined tray and cook on the top shelf of the oven for 40 minutes, breaking it up well with a wooden spoon every 10 minutes. It should have a dark even colour and resemble large coffee granules. Remove and set aside.

3 Meanwhile, pulse the onions, carrot, celery and garlic in a food processor until chopped. Heat the oil in a large non-stick saucepan over a high heat. When hot, add the chopped veg from the processor and cook for 10–15 minutes until starting to caramelise. Sprinkle in the spices and chipotle paste and cook, stirring, for 1 minute.

4 Pour in the stock and add the oregano, kidney beans and tomatoes. Half-fill the empty tomato tins with water, swirl around and pour into the pan. Bring to a gentle simmer. Stir in the roasted mince and cook for 45 minutes, stirring occasionally. Add the peppers and cook gently for 20 minutes or until slightly softened and the mixture is thickened.

5 Spoon the chilli into warmed bowls and top with the avocado, spring onions and coriander. Add a lime wedge to each bowl to serve.

TO FREEZE Once the chilli has thickened, allow to cool then freeze in portions. Defrost fully overnight in the fridge, then reheat in a saucepan over a medium heat until hot all the way through.

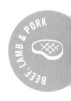

MUSTARD PORK

This classic French-style dish typically has loads of cream and butter. My version uses only a splash of cream and instead the sauce is thickened with a little flour. It's so rich, filling and delicious, it really doesn't taste like diet food at all.

SERVES 2

1 corn-on-the-cob, cut in half
200g fine green beans
2 pork loin steaks (150g each), trimmed of all fat
1 tsp plain flour
1 tsp vegetable oil
250ml fresh chicken stock
2 tsp Dijon mustard
1 tsp wholegrain mustard
75ml single cream
Sea salt and freshly ground black pepper
1 tbsp finely chopped flat-leaf parsley, to finish

1 Bring a medium pan of boiling salted water to the boil, then add the corn cob halves. Bring back to a simmer and cook for 15–20 minutes until tender, adding the green beans to the pan 3–4 minutes before the end.

2 Meanwhile, season the pork steaks all over with salt and pepper, then dust both sides lightly with flour, shaking off any excess.

3 Place a medium non-stick frying pan over a medium-high heat and add the oil. When hot, place the pork steaks in the pan and cook for 2–3 minutes on each side, until golden brown. Remove from the pan and set aside on a plate.

4 Pour the stock into the frying pan, increase the heat to high and let bubble until reduced by half.

5 Once the stock has reduced down in the frying pan, add the mustards and cream and stir well. Cook for 2–3 minutes until the sauce is slightly thickened, then add the pork steaks to the sauce to warm through.

6 Drain the corn and beans. Season them with a little salt and pepper.

7 Taste the mustard sauce and season with salt and pepper if needed. Divide the beans and corn between warmed plates and add the pork steaks. Spoon on the sauce and sprinkle over the chopped parsley.

Per serving: *438 cals*
51g protein   *13g carbs*
19g fat   *6g fibre*

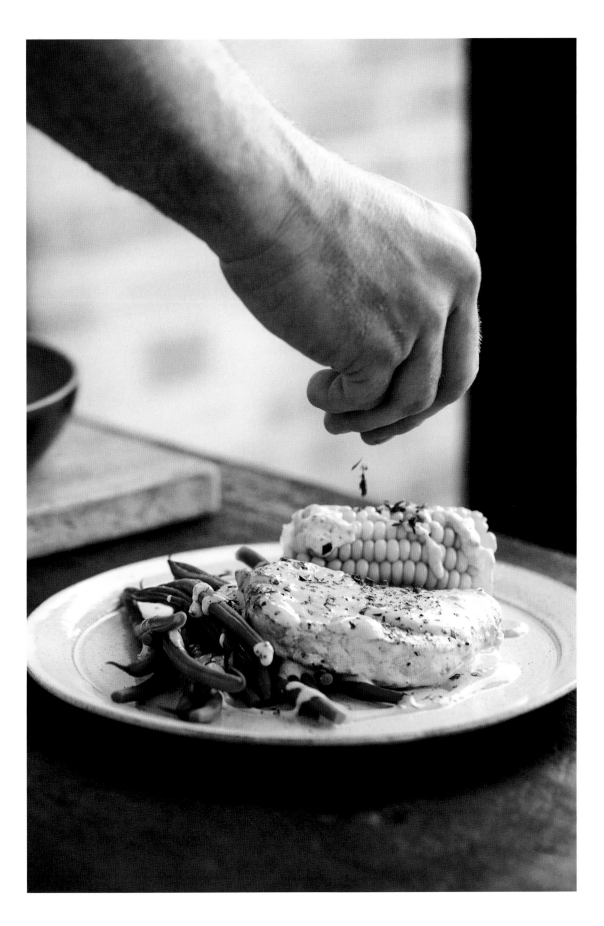

LAMB BHUNA

This dish is all about developing those powerful spice flavourings. Neck of lamb is a great cut of meat to use here, as it has a rich taste and cooks quickly, so you can achieve a similar result to a traditional slow-braised curry. ✳

SERVES 4

1 tbsp vegetable oil
2 onions, finely diced
6 green cardamom pods, lightly crushed
1 cinnamon stick
4 cloves
6 garlic cloves, grated
2.5cm piece fresh ginger, finely grated
3 tsp garam masala
1 heaped tsp ground coriander
1–2 tsp hot chilli powder (depending on how hot you like it)
200ml fresh lamb stock
400g tin chopped tomatoes
800g lamb neck fillet, cut into 3.5cm chunks
1 red pepper
1 green pepper
Sea salt and freshly ground black pepper

To serve
500g cooked brown rice (freshly cooked and drained or 2 pouches)
4 tbsp Greek yoghurt (0% fat)
A small handful of coriander leaves, finely chopped

Per serving: *752 cals*
56g protein   *52g carbs*
34g fat   *6g fibre*

1 Heat the oil in a large heavy-based saucepan over a high heat. When hot, add the onions and cook for 10–15 minutes until starting to turn dark golden. (Add a splash of the stock if they start to catch.)

2 Add the cardamom, cinnamon, cloves, garlic and ginger and cook for 2 minutes. Stir in the ground spices, along with a big pinch of salt, and cook for 30 seconds or until they release their aroma.

3 Pour in the stock, tip in the chopped tomatoes and bring to a gentle simmer. Add the lamb and stir. Cover and cook over a low heat for 40 minutes, stirring occasionally.

4 In the meantime, halve, core and deseed the peppers then cut into 2cm pieces. Add them to the curry, turn up the heat and cook for 10–15 minutes with the lid off, to soften them slightly and reduce the sauce. Remove the whole spices.

5 If using pouches of rice, heat up according to the packet instructions.

6 Serve the curry and rice in warmed bowls with a dollop of yoghurt on the side. Finish with a scattering of coriander.

TO FREEZE Allow the bhuna to cool then freeze in portions. Defrost fully overnight in the fridge, then reheat in a saucepan over a medium heat until hot all the way through.

BEEF, LAMB & PORK

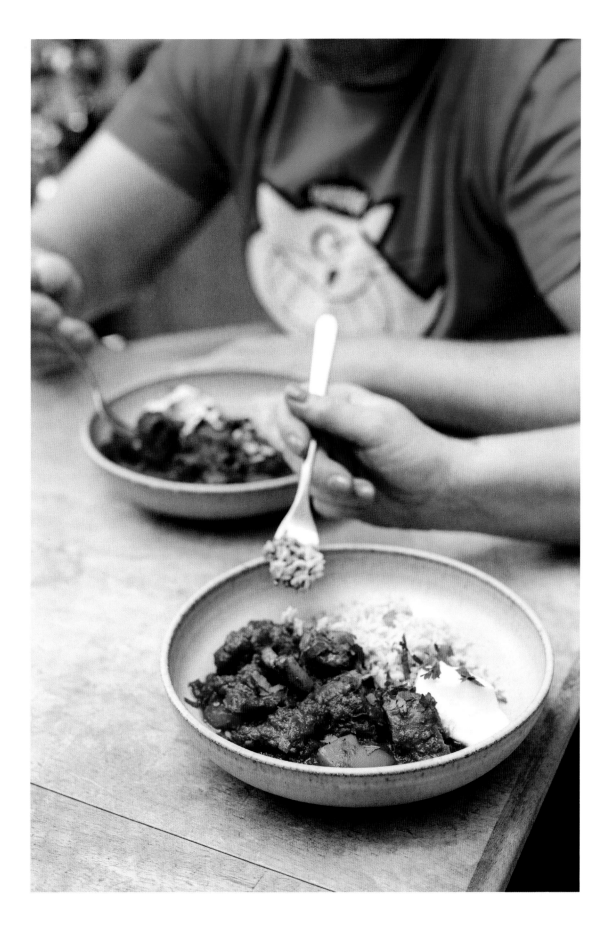

COTTAGE PIE

This is a real childhood favourite of mine – the ultimate in hearty comfort food. A nutmeg-infused sweet potato topping turns your regular cottage pie into something a bit special. ❄

SERVES 8

1kg lean beef mince (5% fat)
2 onions
2 large carrots (250g)
3 celery sticks (150g)
4 garlic cloves, halved
1 tbsp vegetable oil
200ml red wine
1 litre fresh beef stock
2 x 400g tins chopped
    tomatoes
2 tbsp tomato purée
4 sprigs of thyme
2 bay leaves
1 tbsp Worcestershire sauce
250g baby chestnut
    mushrooms, halved
300g frozen peas
Sea salt and freshly ground
    black pepper

For the topping
800g peeled sweet potatoes
600g peeled potatoes
200ml whole milk
¼ nutmeg, finely grated
2 tbsp light vegetable spread
1 tsp Dijon mustard
1 tsp English mustard
50g reduced-fat Cheddar,
    grated
20g Parmesan, freshly grated

Per serving: 552 cals
50g protein   50g carbs
13g fat   10g fibre

1 Preheat the oven to 200°C/Fan 180°C/Gas 6. Line a baking tray with a silicone mat or baking paper.

2 Spread the beef mince out evenly on the lined tray and cook on the top shelf of the oven for 40 minutes, breaking it up well with a wooden spoon every 10 minutes. It should have a dark even colour and resemble large coffee granules. Remove and set aside. Turn off the oven.

3 Meanwhile, quarter the onions and cut the carrots and celery into large chunks. Pulse these veg along with the garlic in a food processor until chopped.

4 Heat the oil in a large non-stick saucepan over a high heat. When hot, add the veg from the food processor and cook for 10–15 minutes, stirring often until they begin to caramelise.

5 Pour in the wine and simmer until reduced by half. Now add the stock, tinned tomatoes, tomato purée and herbs and return to a simmer. Stir in the roasted mince and cook for 30 minutes, stirring occasionally. Add the Worcestershire sauce and mushrooms and cook for a further 30 minutes.

6 Meanwhile, reheat the oven to 200°C/Fan 180°C/Gas 6 and prepare the topping. Cut the sweet potatoes into 3cm dice and the ordinary potatoes into 1.5cm dice. Tip all the potatoes into a large saucepan, cover with cold water and salt the water liberally.

Continued overleaf

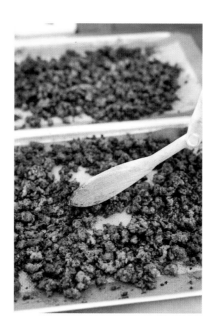

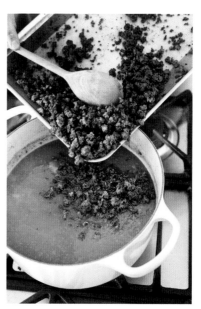

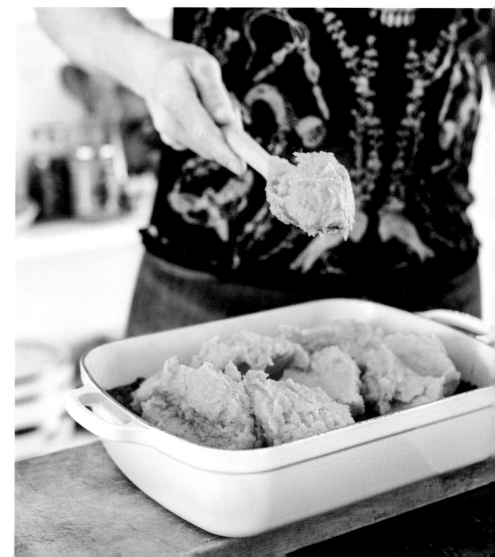

7 Bring to the boil over a high heat, then reduce the heat to a simmer and cook for 15 minutes or until the potatoes are tender. Drain in a colander then pass through a potato ricer back into the pan. Add the milk, nutmeg, vegetable spread, both mustards and a good pinch each of salt and pepper. Mix well.

8 Stir the peas through the mince (removing the thyme and bay leaves if you can find them) and season with salt and pepper to taste.

9 Spoon the mince into a large, fairly deep roasting dish, about 35 x 25cm. Spread the mashed potato in an even layer over the surface and sprinkle with the grated Cheddar and Parmesan. Cook on a high shelf in the oven for 15 minutes and then under the grill for 6–8 minutes or until the cheese is bubbling and browned.

TO FREEZE Leave the pie to cool then pack in a lidded foil container or several containers. Allow to defrost fully in the fridge overnight. Remove the lid(s) and reheat in an oven preheated to 200°C/Fan 180°C/Gas 6 for 20–25 minutes until piping hot all the way through. If the surface appears to be browning too quickly, cover loosely with foil.

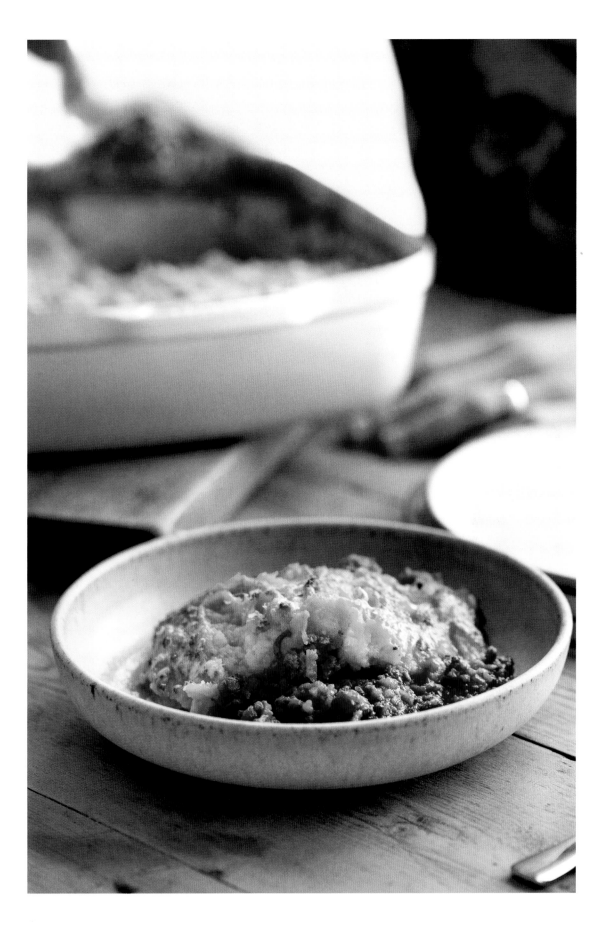

LAMB AND BARLEY STEW

This is a lower-calorie version of a traditional Scotch broth. Pearl barley provides a hearty base, which is offset by the freshness of the peas and mint. ❄

SERVES 4

800g lamb neck fillet
20g plain flour, for dusting
3 tsp vegetable oil
2 leeks (185g), thickly sliced
3 carrots (240g), thickly sliced
4 celery sticks (240g), thickly sliced
2 sprigs of rosemary (or thyme), leaves stripped and roughly chopped
2 bay leaves
1 litre fresh lamb stock
100g pearl barley
240g turnips, peeled and cut into wedges
200g frozen peas
A large handful of mint leaves, finely chopped
Sea salt and freshly ground black pepper

1 Cut the lamb into 2.5cm chunks and season well with salt and pepper. Dust the lamb lightly with flour. Place a large flameproof casserole or non-stick saucepan over a high heat.

2 When the pan is hot, add 1 tsp oil and swirl it around. Add a third of the lamb and cook for about 5 minutes, until browned all over. Transfer to a plate and repeat with the rest of the oil and lamb.

3 Add the leeks and carrots to the pan and cook for 5 minutes, until slightly softened, adding a splash of water if needed. Add the celery, rosemary, bay leaves and stock. Return the lamb to the pan and bring to a simmer.

4 Stir in the pearl barley and add a big pinch each of salt and pepper. Simmer for 20 minutes, then add the turnips and simmer for another 25–30 minutes or until the lamb, turnips and barley are all tender. Add a little more stock or water if you need to.

5 Stir through the peas to defrost and warm through, and fold through the mint. Season with salt and pepper to taste and serve in warmed bowls.

TO FREEZE Allow the stew to cool and then freeze it in portions. Defrost fully overnight in the fridge, then reheat in a saucepan over a medium heat until hot all the way through.

Per serving: *749 cals*
69g protein   *39g carbs*
33g fat   *1g fibre*

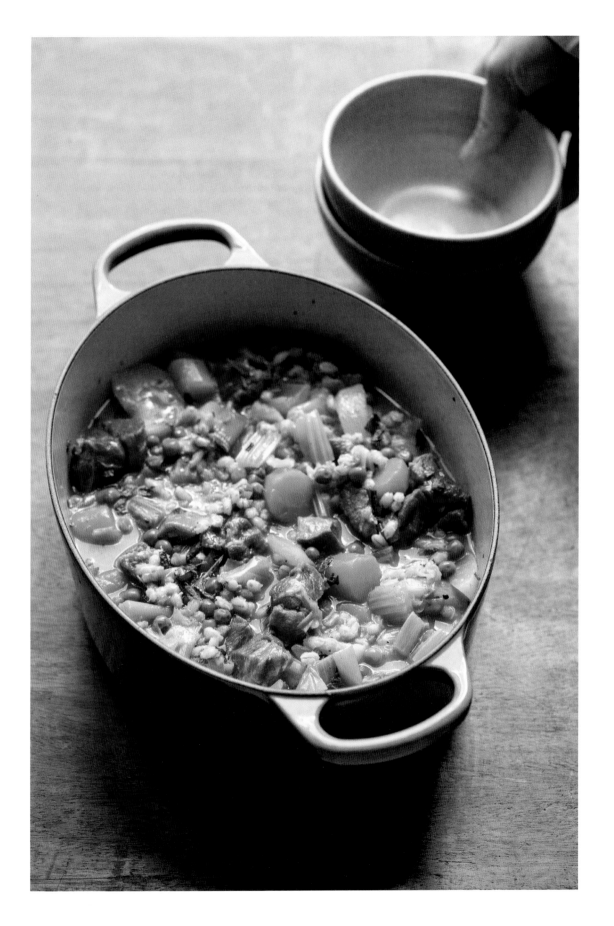

BEEF RAGU WITH PASTA

Everyone has their own version of spag bol, but doing it this way – roasting the mince before you add it to the pan – adds so much extra flavour that once you've tried it, you'll never look back. ❄

SERVES 8

1kg lean beef mince (5% fat)
2 onions
250g carrots
150g celery sticks
4 garlic cloves, halved
1 tbsp vegetable oil
200ml red wine
1 litre fresh beef stock
2 x 400g tins chopped
    tomatoes
2 tbsp sun-dried tomato paste
2 bay leaves
4 sprigs of oregano, leaves
    stripped and finely chopped
4 sprigs of rosemary, leaves
    stripped and finely chopped
2 red peppers, cored,
    deseeded and diced
2 courgettes, diced
300g baby chestnut
    mushrooms, thickly sliced
Sea salt and freshly ground
    black pepper

To serve
80g pasta shells per person
5g Parmesan, finely grated,
    per person

Per serving: 625 cals
54g protein   69g carbs
11g fat   9g fibre

1 Preheat the oven to 200°C/Fan 180°C/Gas 6. Line a baking tray with a silicone mat or baking paper.

2 Spread the beef mince out evenly on the lined tray and cook on the top shelf of the oven for 40 minutes, breaking it up well with a wooden spoon every 10 minutes. It should have a dark even colour and resemble large coffee granules. Remove and set aside.

3 Meanwhile, quarter the onions and chop the carrots and celery into large chunks. Pulse the veg along with the garlic in a food processor until chopped.

4 Heat the oil in a large non-stick saucepan over a high heat. When hot, add the chopped veg from the food processor and cook, stirring often, for 10–15 minutes until starting to caramelise.

5 Pour in the wine and simmer until reduced by half. Now add the stock, tomatoes, tomato paste and herbs and bring to a simmer. Half-fill the empty tomato tins with water, swirl around and pour into the pan. Bring to a gentle simmer. Stir in the roasted mince and cook for 30 minutes, stirring occasionally.

6 Add the peppers, courgettes and mushrooms to the ragu and cook for another 30 minutes.

7 About 10 minutes before serving, bring a large pan of salted water to the boil. Add the pasta and cook, according to the packet instructions, until *al dente*.

8 Drain the pasta and serve with the ragu. Finish with a sprinkling of grated Parmesan.

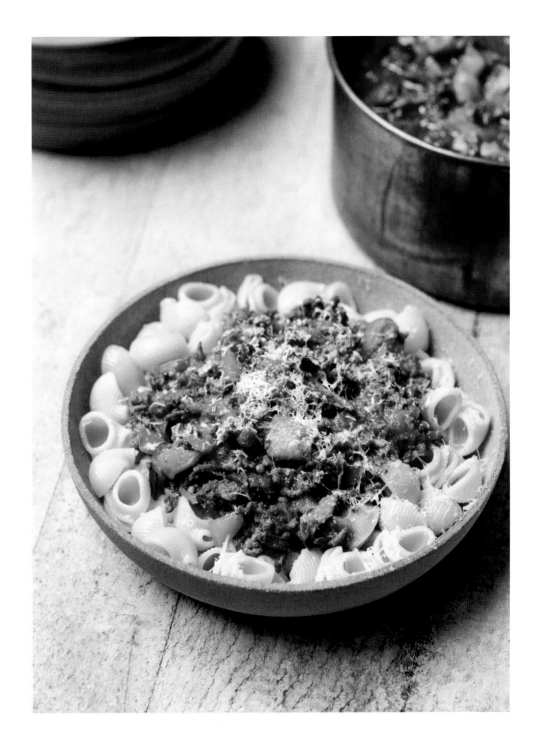

TO FREEZE Allow the ragu to cool and then freeze it in portions. Defrost fully overnight in the fridge, then reheat in a saucepan over a medium heat until hot all the way through.

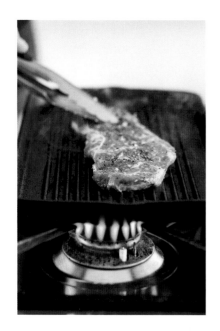

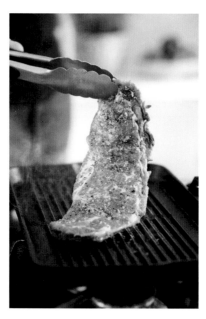

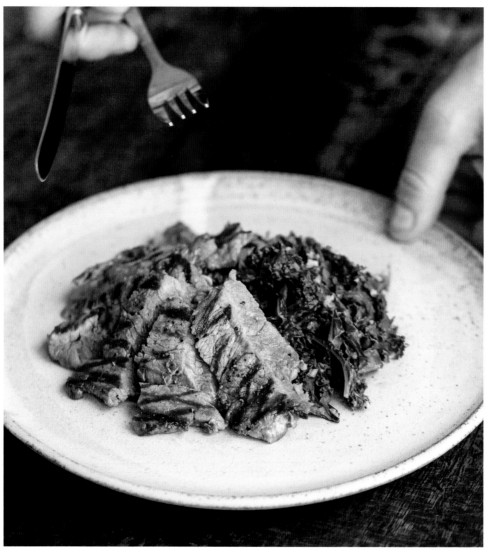

MINUTE STEAKS WITH KALE

Just because you're on a diet, doesn't mean steak night is off the table. This recipe is quick and easy, with maximum tastiness. The anchovies and chillies are great, big flavours that work with the kale – the result is so delicious it almost outshines the beef!

SERVES 2

2 sirloin steaks, trimmed of fat (180g each)
1-cal sunflower oil spray
1 banana shallot, finely diced
2 garlic cloves, finely chopped
250ml fresh beef stock
2 anchovies in oil, drained and finely chopped
1 tsp soy sauce
250g kale, stems removed and roughly shredded
80ml single cream
A pinch of dried chilli flakes
Finely grated zest of ½ lemon
Sea salt and freshly ground black pepper

1 Using a rolling pin, pound each steak out on a board to an even 5mm thickness. Season both sides liberally with salt and pepper.

2 Place a large non-stick frying pan over a medium-high heat. Add a few sprays of oil, then the shallot, and cook for 4 minutes to soften. Add the garlic and cook for 2 minutes, adding a splash of water if the mixture starts to stick.

3 Pour in the stock and let bubble until reduced by half. Meanwhile, place a large non-stick griddle pan over a high heat. Add the anchovies, soy and kale to the shallot and cook for 4 minutes.

4 When the griddle pan is smoking hot, spray each steak with a little oil and place on the griddle. Cook over a very high heat for 1 minute on each side. Remove from the griddle and transfer to a warmed plate to rest.

5 Add the cream, chilli flakes and lemon zest to the kale and cook, stirring, until it is tender and the sauce is thickened. Season with salt and pepper to taste.

6 Spoon the kale onto warmed serving plates, slice the steaks thickly and serve alongside.

Per serving: 435 cals
60g protein   4g carbs
19g fat   5g fibre

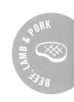

SICHUAN BEEF AND BROCCOLI STIR-FRY

I'm a big fan of Sichuan peppercorns – they have such a distinctive taste. In this ready-in-minutes meal, crunchy fresh green vegetables contrast with the heat from the chillies and salty-sweet soy sauce.

SERVES 2 (generously)

1 tsp vegetable oil
½ tsp Sichuan peppercorns, ground
3 garlic cloves, finely chopped
1 long red chilli, finely sliced
2 dried chillies, broken in half
350g lean beef mince (5% fat)
200g green beans, cut into 2cm pieces
150g tenderstem broccoli, roughly chopped into 2.5cm lengths (any thick stalks halved)
100ml fresh beef stock
1 tbsp soy sauce
Sea salt and freshly ground black pepper

To serve
250g cooked brown rice (freshly cooked and drained or a pouch)
2 spring onions, green part only, finely shredded

1 Place a large non-stick wok over a high heat. When it is smoking hot, swirl in the oil, add the Sichuan peppercorns and garlic and stir-fry for 1–2 minutes.

2 Toss in the fresh and dried chillies and cook for 30 seconds. Now add the mince and stir-fry for 3–4 minutes or until it is richly browned all over.

3 Add the green beans, broccoli, stock and soy sauce and stir-fry for 2–4 minutes, until the greens are tender and the stock is totally reduced. Meanwhile, if using a pouch of rice, heat it up according to the packet instructions.

4 Season the stir-fry with salt and pepper to taste. Serve in warmed bowls with the cooked rice. Finish with a scattering of shredded spring onions.

BONUS This quick meal is loaded with protein and vitamin C. Broccoli also has lots of anti-inflammatory nutrients to help boost your post-workout recovery.

Per serving: *497 cals*
53g protein   *42g carbs*
11g fat   *9g fibre*

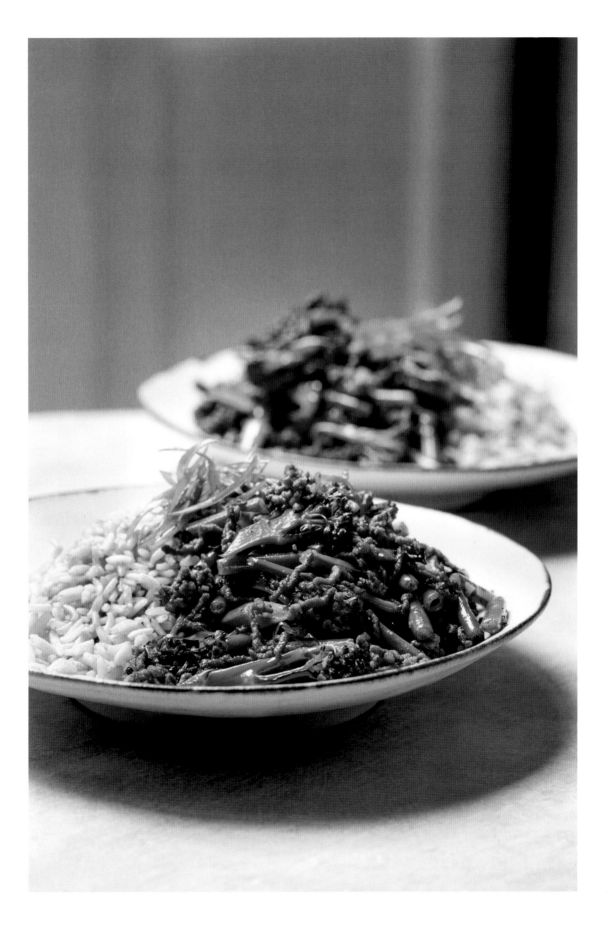

PORK LOIN WITH CELERIAC, GARLIC AND CIDER

Pork and cider is a traditional West Country pairing that is hard to beat. With the addition of earthy celeriac, this is a great dish for a winter day or as an alternative to a Sunday roast.

SERVES 4

1kg boneless pork loin, trimmed of all fat, at room temperature
2 tsp olive oil
300g banana shallots, halved lengthways
300ml cider
500ml fresh chicken stock, plus a little extra if needed
1 head of garlic, cloves separated (unpeeled)
700g peeled celeriac, cut into 2.5cm cubes
2 bay leaves
10 sprigs of thyme
150g frozen peas
Sea salt and freshly ground black pepper

1 Preheat the oven to 180°C/Fan 160°C/Gas 4. Season the pork generously all over with salt and pepper. Place a large non-stick frying pan over a high heat and add 1 tsp oil. When hot, add the pork to the pan and brown well on all sides to enhance the flavour; this should take about 10 minutes.

2 Remove the pork from the pan and set aside. Add the remaining oil to the pan then add the shallots, cut side down. Cook for 2–3 minutes on each side until golden brown. Remove the shallots from the pan.

3 Add the cider to the pan to deglaze, scraping up all the brown bits from the base. Let the cider bubble to reduce by half, then pour in the stock. Stir well and simmer until the liquor is reduced by half again.

4 Put the shallots, garlic cloves, celeriac, bay leaves and thyme into a roasting tin. Place the pork on top and pour over the reduced liquor. Season the veg with salt and pepper and cover the roasting tin with foil.

5 Cook in the oven for 30 minutes, then remove the foil and roast for a further 15 minutes. Take the pork out of the pan and leave to rest in a warm place, covered with foil, while you finish cooking the veg.

6 Turn the oven up to 200°C/Fan 180°C/Gas 6. Return the roasting tin of veg to the oven to cook for a further 20 minutes, adding more stock if it becomes too dry. Remove from the oven and stir through the frozen peas to warm through. Carve the pork and serve with the vegetables, spooning over the pan juices.

Per serving: *532 cals*
76g protein   *12g carbs*
15g fat   *12g fibre*

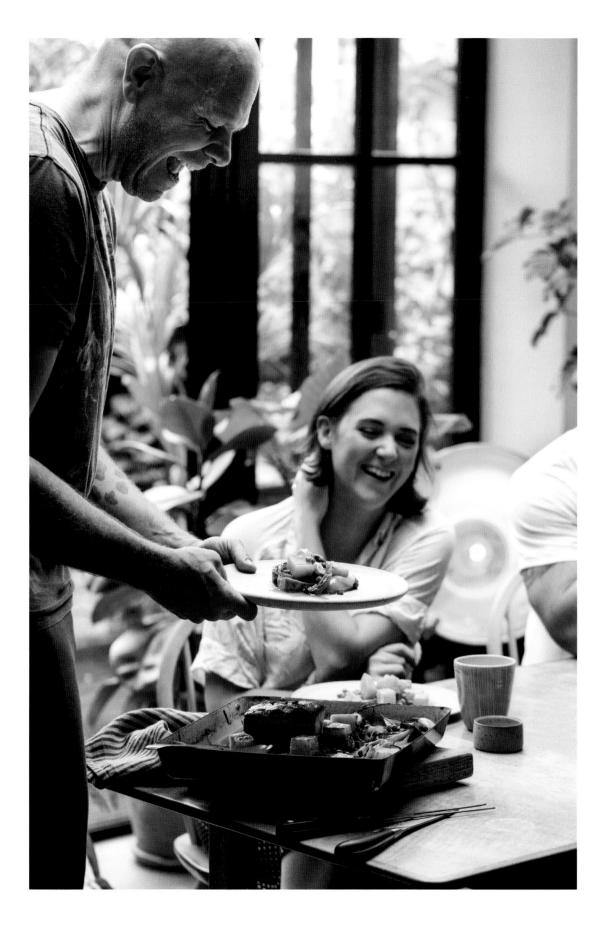

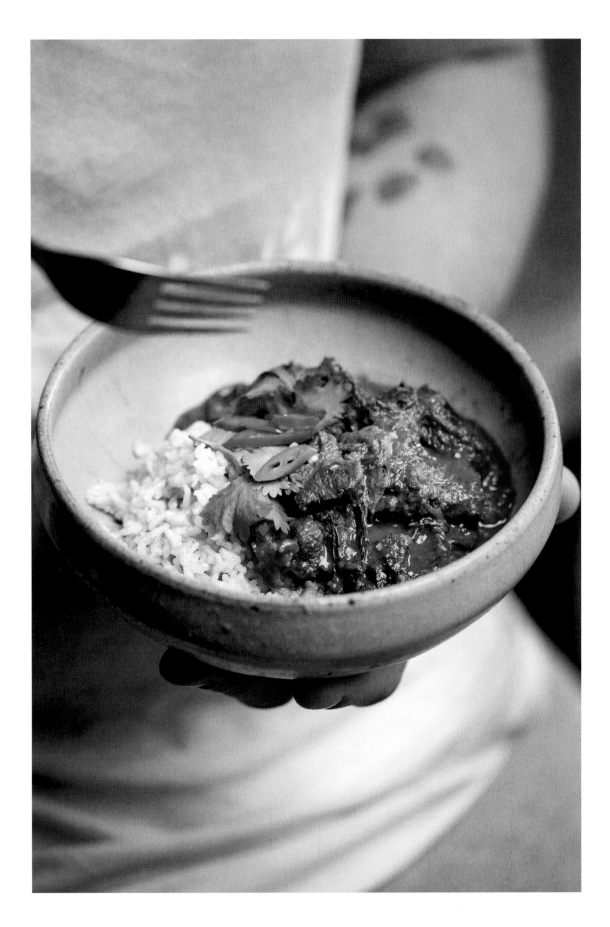

MALAYSIAN-STYLE BEEF CURRY

Here, galangal, tamarind and lemongrass introduce more subtle flavours than the often fiery heat of a classic Indian curry. Give it a try to make a change from your usual curry. ❄

SERVES 4

650g lean stewing beef
1 tbsp vegetable oil
1 litre fresh beef stock
1 cinnamon stick
2 star anise
2 kaffir lime leaves
150ml tinned coconut milk
1 tbsp tamarind paste
Sea salt and freshly ground
    black pepper

For the spice paste
8 shallots, quartered
4 garlic cloves, peeled
2 dried chillies, stalks removed
2 long red chillies, deseeded
2.5cm piece fresh ginger, diced
2.5cm piece fresh galangal,
    diced
2 lemongrass stems, coarse
    layers removed, chopped
1 tsp ground turmeric

To finish and serve
500g cooked brown rice
    (freshly cooked and drained
    or 2 pouches)
A handful of coriander leaves
1 long red chilli, finely sliced

Per serving: *613 cals*
66g protein   *42g carbs*
19g fat   *3g fibre*

1 First, prepare the spice paste: put all the ingredients into a food processor along with 1 tsp salt and blend until smooth, adding a splash of water if needed.

2 Cut the beef into 2.5cm cubes. Place a large non-stick saucepan over a high heat and add the oil. When hot, add the spice paste and cook, stirring, for 1 minute or until fragrant.

3 Add the beef and cook, stirring regularly, for 5 minutes until starting to brown. Add the stock, cinnamon, star anise and lime leaves. Bring to a low simmer, cover and cook gently for 45 minutes, stirring occasionally. Remove the lid and cook for a further 20 minutes or until the sauce is thickened and the beef is tender.

4 Increase the heat, stir in the coconut milk and tamarind paste and cook for a further 5 minutes. Meanwhile, if using pouches of rice, heat up according to the packet instructions. Season the curry with salt and pepper to taste and discard the cinnamon stick and star anise.

5 Divide the rice and curry between warmed bowls and top with coriander leaves and chilli slices to serve.

TO FREEZE Let the curry cool then freeze in portions. Defrost fully overnight in the fridge, then reheat in a pan over a medium heat until hot all the way through.

 BONUS Lean stewing steak is high in protein and very low in saturated fat – less than 2% – compared with other cuts of beef.

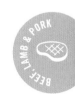

217

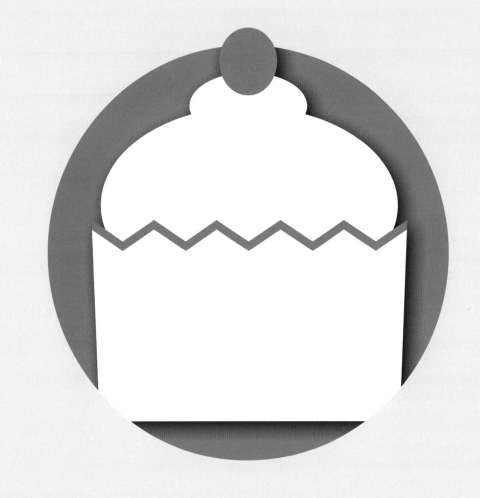

8 SWEET

I WONDER HOW MANY OF YOU turned straight to this chapter? I get it. Losing weight and exercising regularly is hard work. It's about making big long-term changes to your lifestyle and sometimes that can feel overwhelming. Cakes, chocolate and puddings may be some of the hardest things to give up. But if this is a really tough one for you, then there's no point totally denying yourself. It'll only make you want it more. And before you know it, you'll succumb to a packet of biscuits.

You can still treat yourself from time to time, just be a bit wiser with your choices – and don't make it an everyday occurrence. If you're eating properly balanced meals, you should be satisfied, but if you're craving something sweet, choose puddings with fruit and nuts so you get in some goodness at the same time, and avoid desserts that are high in added sugars.

Greek yoghurt is a great ingredient to work into your desserts, as it has a lovely, sharp tang and a rich, creamy texture, and it's high in protein – much higher than other yoghurts. Try it in the blackberry fool on page 220, lemon and blueberry yoghurt pots on page 222 or the panna cottas on page 225.

An ingredient I've come to favour recently is chia seeds. They are rich in healthy omega-3 fatty acids as well as being high in protein and fibre, but I particularly like them for the texture they develop. The seeds are crunchy, but the longer you leave them to soak, the smoother the resulting consistency. Try them in the chocolate chia puddings on page 226, which have an intense chocolate flavour and a thick, rich texture – you really won't believe this dessert is as healthy as it is. Oats are another good way to get in extra nutrients, and they add a nutty crunch to the berry crumble on page 228.

For those times when only cake will do, bake a pear and ginger loaf cake or some chocolate and raspberry cupcakes (see pages 234 and 237). Made with wholemeal flour and minimal sugars, both are healthier than regular versions, but they're still high in flavour.

If you need a quick boost at any time of the day, the energy balls on pages 238–243 are packed with all the good stuff: nuts, oats, dried fruits, spices and delicious all-natural flavourings. These are so much better for you than shop-bought energy bars, and will save you money too. They'll last for quite a while in the fridge, so make a batch in case of emergencies.

You don't want to feel like you're missing out on the things you enjoy when you're dieting. It's OK to have a sweet treat every now and then – just make a real celebration of it, and then get yourself back on track.

BLACKBERRY AND YOGHURT FOOL

The two types of yoghurt in this fruity fool provide the perfect consistency when mixed together, but if you like you can use all fat-free yoghurt. Diced Granny Smith apples in the compote provide a lovely, sharp acidity that works really well alongside the fiery ginger.

SERVES 4

400g Greek yoghurt (0% fat)
300g full-fat Greek yoghurt
1 vanilla pod, split and seeds scraped
2 tbsp granulated sweetener

For the fruit compote
2 Granny Smith apples, peeled and diced (300g prepared weight)
300g blackberries (fresh or frozen)
½ tsp ground cardamom
2 balls (40g) preserved stem ginger in syrup, drained and finely chopped
2 tbsp granulated sweetener
100ml water

To finish
15g nibbed pistachio nuts, roughly pulsed in a mini food processor or finely chopped

1 For the compote, put all of the ingredients into a small saucepan and bring to a steady simmer over a medium-high heat. Cook for 8–10 minutes or until the apples are tender and the compote is syrupy. Leave to cool completely.

2 Put both yoghurts into a large bowl, add the vanilla seeds and sweetener and whisk until well combined.

3 Fold half the fruit compote gently into the yoghurt mixture until rippled through. Spoon into serving bowls, top with the remaining compote and sprinkle with the pistachios to serve.

BONUS Greek yoghurt is strained to give it its thick consistency. As a result it contains twice as much protein as regular yoghurt – a real benefit as protein is vital for strengthening your muscles and helping them recover after exercise.

Per serving: *253 cals*
19g protein   *28g carbs*
6g fat   *4g fibre*

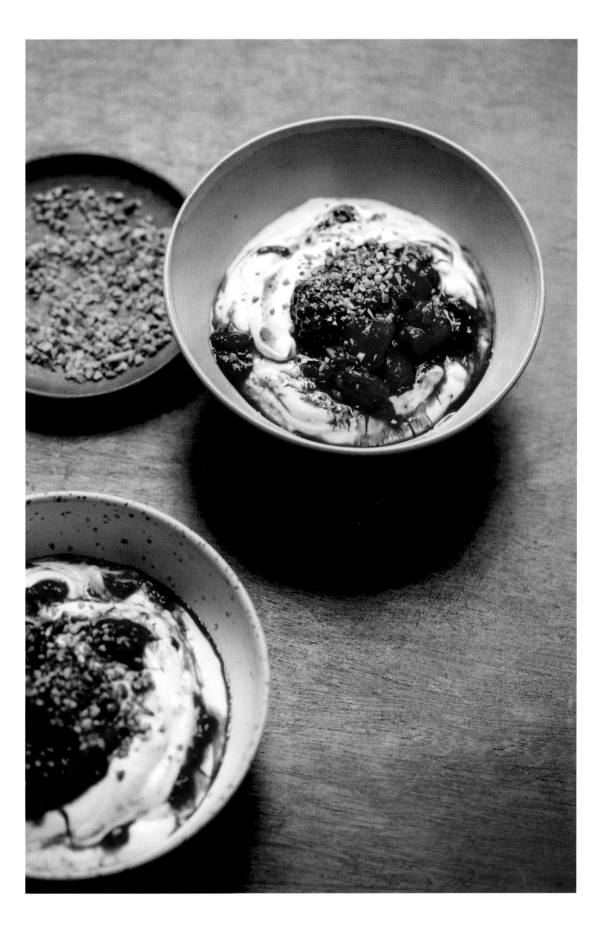

LEMON AND BLUEBERRY YOGHURT POTS

Blueberries are a massive thing in my house and we usually have loads of them around because Little Man loves them – they even get eaten with his fish fingers! This is a great way to use them in a proper recipe. ♡

SERVES 4

150g blueberries
Finely grated zest of ½ lemon
1 vanilla pod, split and seeds scraped
40ml water
2 tsp granulated sweetener
450g lemon Greek-style yoghurt (0% fat)
3 reduced-calorie rich tea biscuits (26g)
1 tsp cornflour, mixed with 1 tsp water
½ ready-made individual meringue (18g), lightly crushed

1 Put the blueberries into a small saucepan with the lemon zest, vanilla seeds, water and sweetener. Bring to a simmer over a medium-high heat and let simmer for 5 minutes.

2 Meanwhile, in a small bowl, whisk the lemon yoghurt until smooth. Crumble the biscuits roughly into a separate bowl.

3 Once the blueberries have cooked down, stir in the cornflour paste and cook, stirring, until thickened. Remove from the heat and leave to cool.

4 When the blueberries have cooled completely, add them to the lemon yoghurt and mix lightly until swirled through.

5 Put a generous spoonful of the blueberry yoghurt into each of 4 serving glasses (150ml capacity) and layer the crumbled biscuits on top. Spoon on the remaining yoghurt mixture, top with the crushed meringue and serve immediately.

Per serving: *128 cals*
8g protein   *21g carbs*
1g fat   *1g fibre*

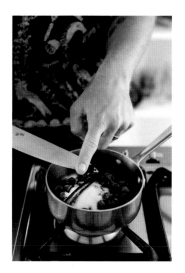

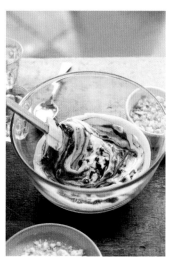

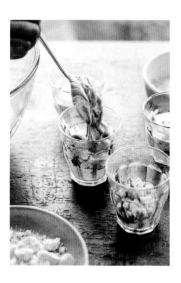

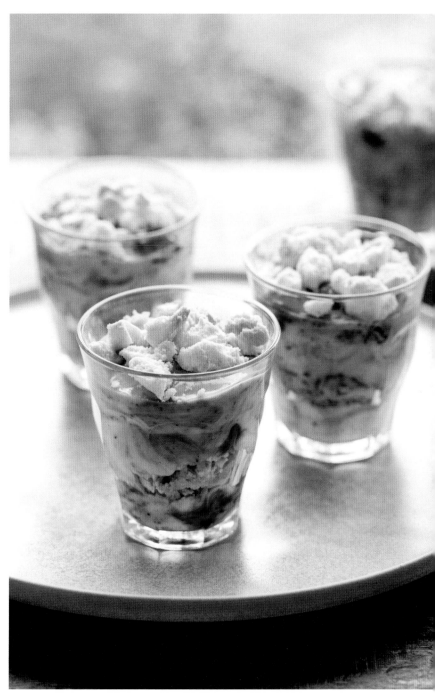

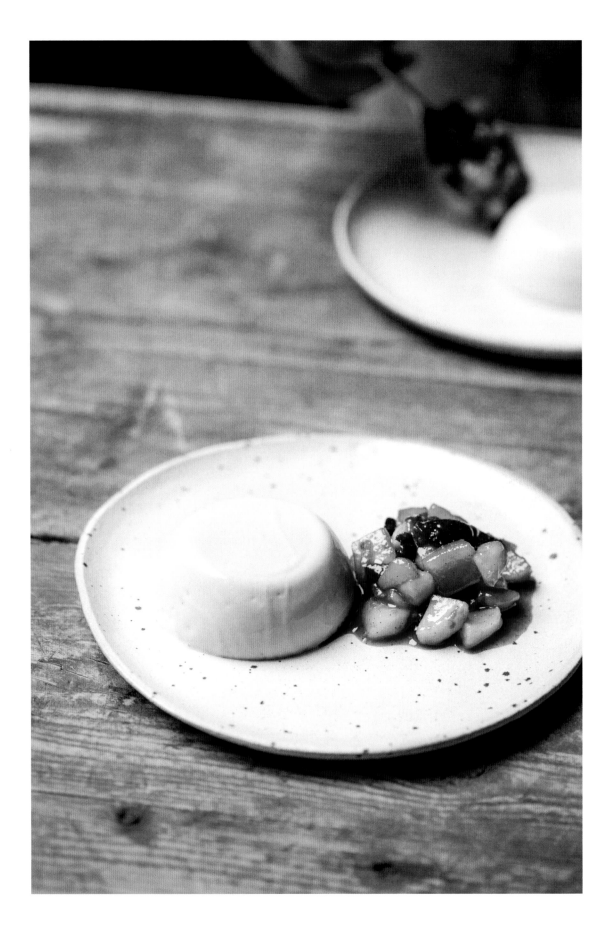

EARL GREY PANNA COTTAS

A rich and creamy dessert will always taste like a calorific treat, but these are made with Greek yoghurt, keeping them lower in fat and calories than traditional panna cotta. If you're not a fan of Earl Grey, swap it out for a flavour you like – try the seeds from a vanilla pod or 1 tsp instant coffee granules.

SERVES 4

2 sheets of leaf gelatine
200ml whole milk
100ml single cream
2 Earl Grey tea bags
2 tbsp granulated sweetener
250g Greek yoghurt (0% fat)

For the fruit compote
1 orange
2 tbsp Pedro Ximénez sherry
½ vanilla pod, split and seeds scraped
100ml water
150g ripe pear, peeled and roughly diced
150g Granny Smith apple, peeled and roughly diced
50g Agen prunes, quartered

Per serving: 194 cals
11g protein   19g carbs
7g fat   2g fibre

1 In a shallow dish, soak the gelatine in cold water to cover for 5 minutes. Meanwhile, pour the milk and cream into a small saucepan, add the tea bags and bring to a very gentle simmer. Stir in the sweetener, then take off the heat and let steep for 5 minutes or until well infused with the Earl Grey (taste to check).

2 Bring the infused creamy milk back to a simmer, then take off the heat and remove the tea bags, squeezing out all the liquid. Immediately drain the gelatine, squeeze out excess water and add to the hot creamy milk, stirring to dissolve. Leave to cool slightly.

3 In a bowl, lightly whisk the yoghurt. Add the infused mixture and whisk again until smooth. Pour into four ramekins (150ml capacity) and refrigerate for 2 hours to set.

4 Meanwhile, prepare the fruit compote. Pare 3 strips of orange zest and place them in a small saucepan along with the juice from the orange, the sherry, vanilla pod and seeds and the water. Bring to a simmer and let bubble to reduce by half. Add the pear, apple and prunes and simmer gently for 5 minutes or until the fruit is tender and the liquid is syrupy. Remove from the heat and discard the orange zest and vanilla pod.

5 When the panna cottas are set, gently press them around the edges to release them from the ramekins and carefully turn out on to serving plates. Serve with the compote.

SWEET

CHOCOLATE CHIA PUDDINGS

Chia seeds are a great way of thickening and enriching a dish. Dark chocolate adds a sophisticated note, while shop-bought custard ensures this deliciously rich and creamy pudding is quick and easy to make. ♡

SERVES 4

500g light custard
100ml whole milk
1 vanilla pod, split and seeds scraped
30g good-quality cocoa powder
50g dark chocolate (70% cocoa solids), roughly chopped
1 tbsp granulated sweetener
4 tbsp chia seeds
180g raspberries

1 Pour the custard and milk into a medium saucepan and add the vanilla pod and seeds, cocoa powder, dark chocolate and sweetener.

2 Place over a medium-low heat and heat slowly, whisking gently until the chocolate is completely melted – this will only take a couple of minutes. Remove from the heat and discard the vanilla pod.

3 Add the chia seeds to the chocolate mixture and whisk again until well combined.

4 Divide half the raspberries between 4 small jars or glasses (about 280ml capacity). Spoon the chia mixture into the glasses and place in the fridge for 2 hours to chill.

5 Pile the remaining raspberries on top of the puddings to serve.

 BONUS Chia seeds are full of healthy omega-3 fatty acids, protein and fibre – which all help stave off hunger. And dark chocolate contains antioxidants which help you to recover after a workout.

SWEET

Per serving: *301 cals*
11g protein   *33g carbs*
13g fat   *8g fibre*

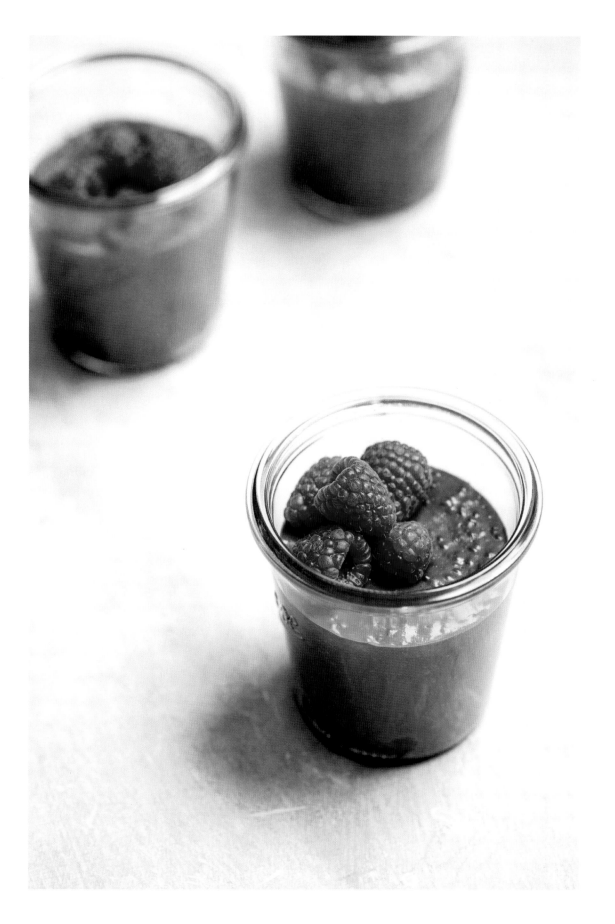

MIXED BERRY CRUMBLE

You can't beat a classic fruit crumble to round off a meal when it's cold outside, and this one is big enough to serve a crowd. If you are making it for fewer people, simply freeze the rest for another day. The walnuts and oats in the topping give it a great crunchy texture. ♡ ❄

SERVES 12

3 Granny Smith apples, peeled and grated (480g prepared weight)
3 small Bramley apples, peeled and cut into 2cm dice (480g prepared weight)
800g frozen mixed berries
1 tsp ground mixed spice
½ tsp ground cardamom
½ tsp ground cinnamon
3 tbsp granulated sweetener
Juice of 1 lemon
Juice of 1 orange

For the topping
250g rolled oats
3 tbsp granulated sweetener
100g wholemeal flour
150g walnuts, roughly ground (in a mini food processor)
100g light vegetable spread, in small pieces

1 Preheat the oven to 200°C/Fan 180°C/Gas 6.

2 Put the apples and berries into a large (30 x 25cm) roasting dish. Sprinkle over the spices, sweetener and the lemon and orange juices. Mix all the ingredients together well.

3 For the topping, in a large bowl, mix together the rolled oats, sweetener, wholemeal flour and ground walnuts. Add the vegetable spread and rub in well with your fingertips.

4 Spread the oat and nut mixture over the fruit and cook in the oven for 45–60 minutes, until the apples are tender and the topping is golden and crispy.

TO FREEZE Allow the berry crumble to cool, then freeze in two-portion foil trays with cardboard lids. Defrost fully in the fridge overnight. Remove the lids, then reheat in the oven preheated to 200°C/Fan 180°C/Gas 6 for 25–30 minutes until piping hot. If the surface appears to be browning too quickly, cover loosely with foil.

SWEET

Per serving: *298 cals*
7g protein   *34g carbs*
14g fat   *6g fibre*

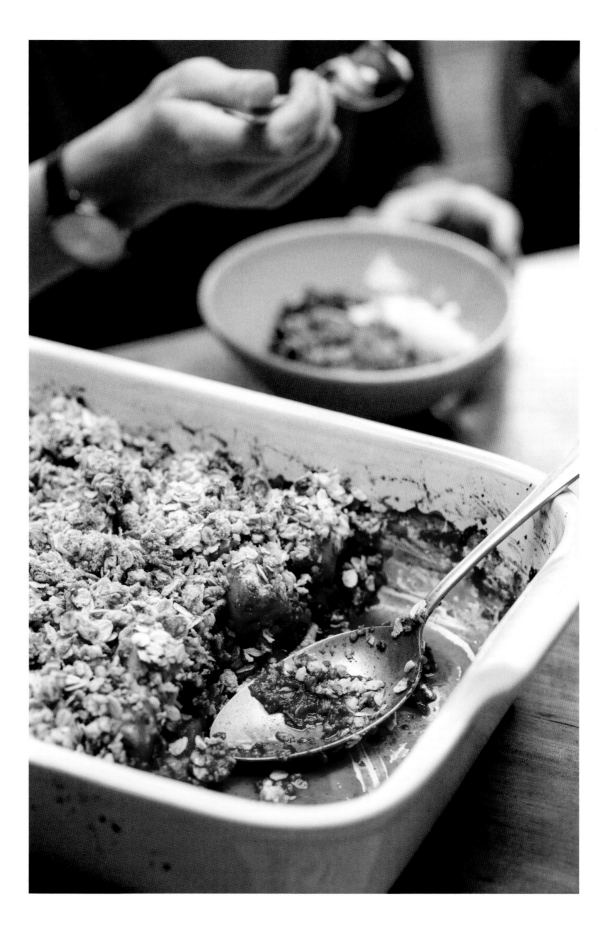

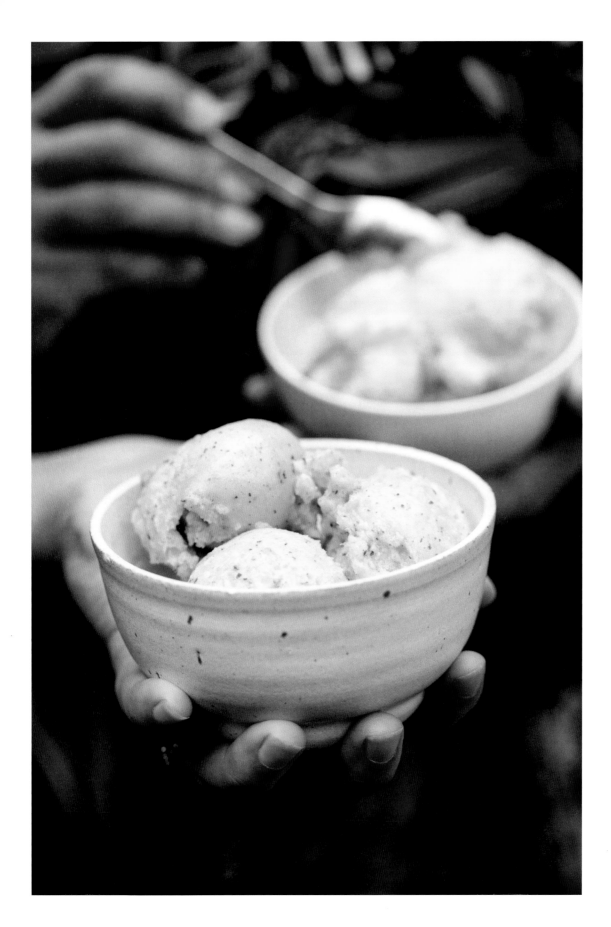

MELON AND MINT SORBET

This melon and mint sorbet is such a special way of putting together a dessert with almost zero guilt. It tastes clean, crisp and refreshing – and it's effortless to make. Use a really sweet, ripe melon for maximum flavour. ♡ ❅

SERVES 4

750g peeled and deseeded ripe cantaloupe melon
100ml apple and elderflower juice
40ml maple syrup
50ml water
2 tbsp granulated sweetener
Juice of 1 lime
2 small handfuls of mint leaves

1 Cut the melon into 2.5cm chunks and freeze on a tray until solid.

2 Pour the apple and elderflower juice into a small saucepan and add the maple syrup, water, sweetener, lime juice and half the mint leaves. Bring to a gentle simmer over a medium-high heat and cook gently for 5 minutes.

3 Take the pan off the heat and leave the mixture to cool and infuse. Once cooled, strain and discard the mint leaves.

4 Put the frozen melon into a food processor along with the cooled syrup and remaining mint leaves. Blitz until smooth, then spoon the sorbet into bowls and enjoy immediately.

TO FREEZE Transfer the sorbet to a suitable container and freeze. Allow to soften at room temperature for 10 minutes or so before serving.

Per serving: *82 cals*
1g protein *17g carbs*
0g fat *13g fibre*

FUDGY CHOCOLATE BROWNIES

Black beans give these brownies a rich, gooey texture and an inviting deep colour. They taste totally lush and are worth every calorie! Just keep a close eye on them in the oven, as they're liable to become dry if overcooked. ♡ ❄

MAKES 9

400g tin black beans, drained and rinsed (235g drained weight)
80g light vegetable spread
4 large free-range eggs
60g good-quality cocoa powder, plus 1 tsp to finish
50g ground almonds
1 tbsp vanilla extract
40ml maple syrup
1 tsp instant coffee granules
4 tbsp granulated sweetener
60g dark chocolate chips

1 Preheat the oven to 180°C/Fan 160°C/Gas 4. Line a 20cm square baking tin with baking paper.

2 Put the black beans and vegetable spread into a food processor and blend until smooth. Add the eggs and blend again briefly, until well combined. Transfer the mixture to a large bowl.

3 Add the cocoa powder, ground almonds, vanilla extract, maple syrup, coffee granules, sweetener and half the chocolate chips. Whisk to combine evenly.

4 Pour the mixture into the lined baking tin and sprinkle the remaining chocolate chips over the surface. Bake on the middle shelf of the oven for 18–20 minutes until just firm to the touch.

5 Remove from the oven and leave to cool slightly before carefully lifting the brownie out of the tin and cutting it into squares. Enjoy while still warm, sprinkled with a little sifted cocoa if you like.

TO FREEZE Allow to cool completely then wrap the brownie squares in foil and transfer to a rigid container. Defrost at room temperature.

 BONUS Using black beans means you need a lot less fat than regular brownies call for. The beans also add extra fibre and protein.

Per brownie: *209 cals*
9g protein   *14g carbs*
12g fat   *4g fibre*

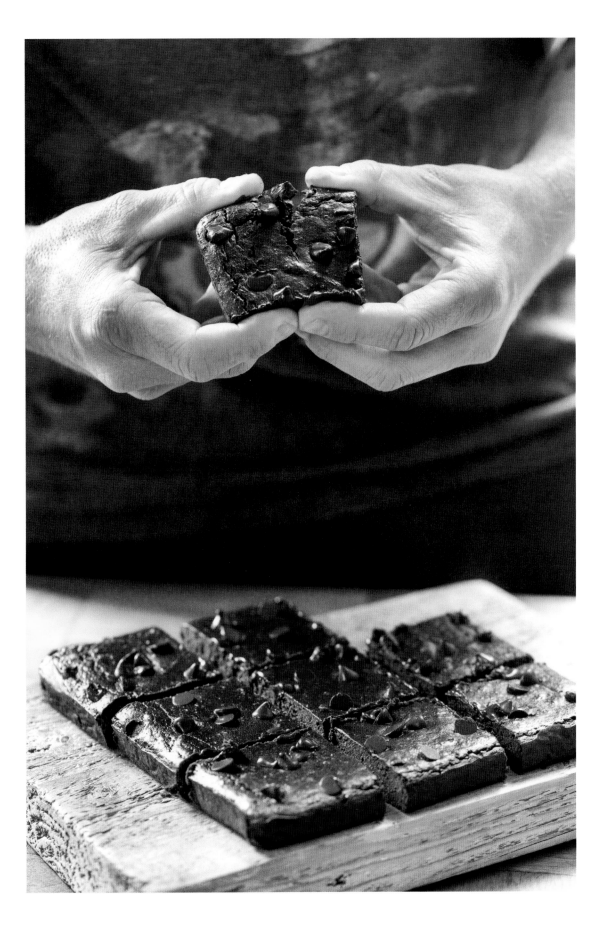

PEAR AND GINGER LOAF CAKE

Filling, robust and super-tasty, this is everything you want from a fruity loaf cake. Eat it while still a little warm from the oven, or grill slices and top them with cottage cheese. It's a perfect combination of sweet and savoury. ♡ ❄

MAKES 8 SLICES

1-cal sunflower oil spray
125g light vegetable spread
2 tbsp treacle
2 tbsp granulated sweetener
75ml whole milk
2 large free-range eggs
50g preserved stem ginger
    in syrup, drained and finely
    chopped
200g self-raising wholemeal
    flour
1 tsp baking powder
1 tbsp ground ginger
1 tsp ground cinnamon
1 tsp ground allspice
2 ripe pears, peeled, cored
    and grated (200g prepared
    weight)

1 Preheat the oven to 200°C/Fan 180°C/Gas 6. Spray a 450g (1lb) loaf tin with a few sprays of oil and line with baking paper.

2 Put the vegetable spread, treacle and sweetener into a medium bowl. Using an electric hand mixer, beat until well combined.

3 Add the milk, eggs, chopped stem ginger, flour, baking powder and spices to the mixture and beat again until smooth. Using a large metal spoon or spatula, fold in the grated pears.

4 Transfer the mixture to the lined loaf tin and spread evenly. Bake for 35–40 minutes until a skewer inserted into the middle comes out clean, indicating the cake is cooked.

5 Remove the cake from the oven and leave in the tin for 5 minutes, then turn out onto a wire rack and leave to cool slightly. Serve cut into slices, ideally while still slightly warm.

TO FREEZE Cut the cake into slices and place a piece of greaseproof paper in between each one. Freeze in a ziplock bag. Defrost at room temperature.

Per slice: *202 cals*
5g protein   *27g carbs*
8g fat   *1g fibre*

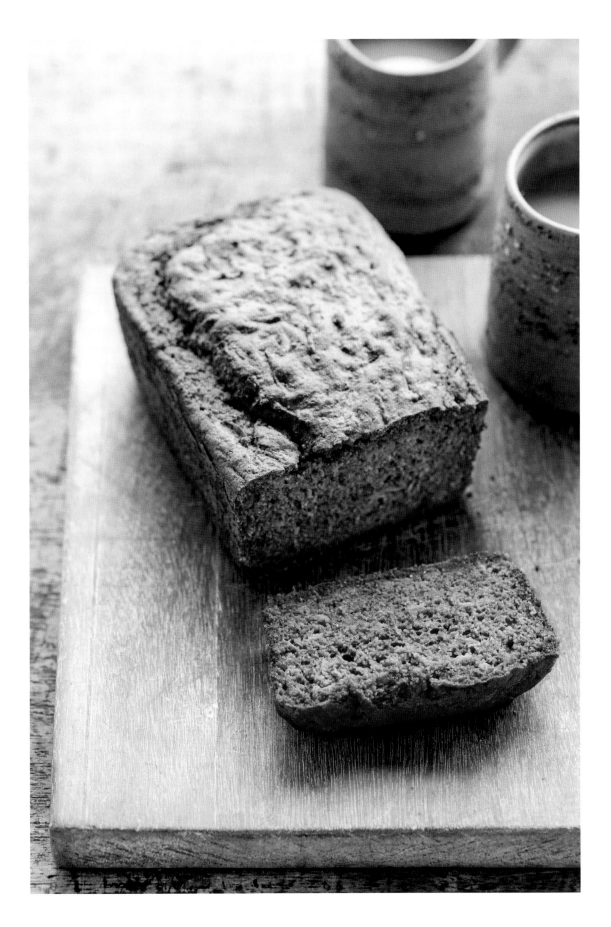

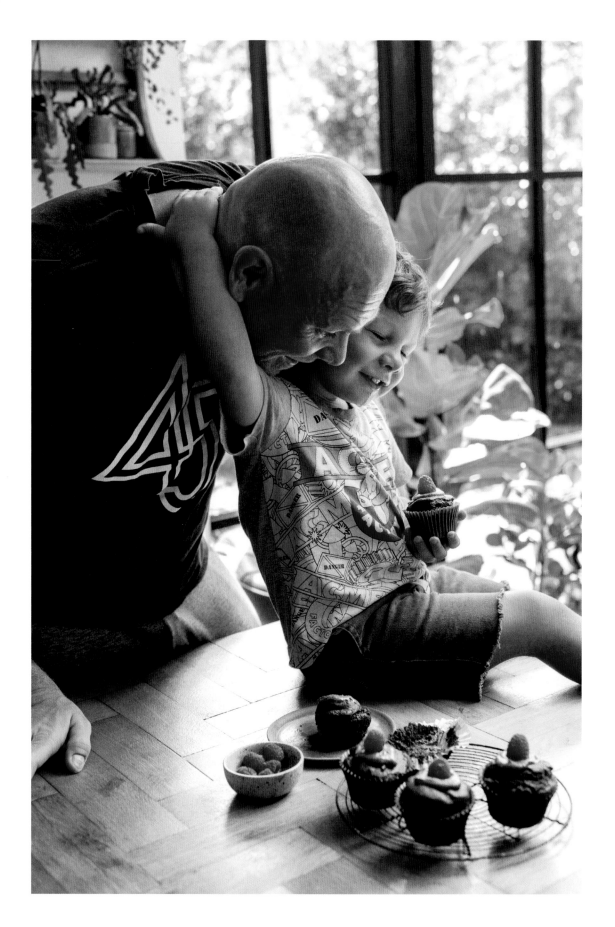

CHOCOLATE AND RASPBERRY CUPCAKES

Fresh raspberries give these irresistible chocolate cupcakes little pockets of fruity freshness. The icing makes them feel like a real treat but they are still amazingly relatively low in calories. ♡

MAKES 12

1-cal sunflower oil spray
150g self-raising wholemeal
    flour
85g good-quality cocoa
    powder
2 tsp baking powder
1 tsp instant coffee granules
4 tbsp granulated sweetener
A pinch of sea salt
50g light vegetable spread,
    melted
1 tbsp vanilla extract
150ml whole milk
120g Greek yoghurt (0% fat)
2 large free-range eggs,
    lightly beaten
60ml maple syrup
24 raspberries (100g)

For the chocolate icing
30g light vegetable spread
1 tbsp cocoa powder
20g icing sugar

To finish
12 raspberries (50g)

1 Preheat the oven to 180°C/Fan 160°C/Gas 4. Line a 12-cup muffin tray with paper muffin cases and spray the inside of each one with a spray of oil.

2 Put all of the dry ingredients into a medium bowl and whisk lightly to mix.

3 In a large bowl, whisk together the melted vegetable spread, vanilla extract, milk, yoghurt, eggs and maple syrup until well combined.

4 Add one-third of the flour mix to the whisked mixture and whisk until smooth. Repeat this twice more to incorporate the rest of the flour mix.

5 Place 2 raspberries in the bottom of each cupcake case. Spoon in the cake mixture, dividing it evenly. Bake on the middle shelf of the oven for 20 minutes, or until a cocktail stick inserted into the centre comes out clean.

6 Remove from the oven and let the cupcakes cool slightly in their tray for 5 minutes, then transfer them to a wire rack and leave to cool completely.

7 Meanwhile, to make the chocolate icing, mix the vegetable spread, cocoa and icing sugar together in a small bowl until smooth. Spoon a small dollop of icing on top of each cake and finish with a raspberry.

Per cupcake: *150 cals*
6g protein   *16g carbs*
6g fat   *3g fibre*

SWEET

237

CARROT CAKE ENERGY BALLS

These have all the flavours of my favourite cake rolled up into tasty bite-sized portions. The sweetness comes from the dates, which are a great natural alternative for sugar if you have a sweet tooth. ♡ ❄

MAKES 20

200g Medjool dates, pitted
   and roughly chopped
100ml boiling water
200g carrots, grated
50g rolled oats
50g desiccated coconut, plus
   an extra 40g to finish
80g walnuts, toasted
80g pecan nuts, toasted
1 tsp ground cinnamon
1 tsp ground mixed spice
1 tbsp vanilla extract

1 Place the dates in a heatproof bowl and pour on the boiling water. Cover and leave to soak for 10 minutes.

2 Put the rest of the ingredients into a food processor. Drain the dates in a sieve over a bowl to save the water, then add them to the processor and pulse until well combined. If the mixture is too dry, add a little of the date water and pulse again.

3 Divide the mixture into 20 balls, each a bit larger than a golf ball. Roll each ball well to create an even shape and then roll in the extra desiccated coconut to coat.

4 Place on a tray and refrigerate for 1 hour before serving. Store any uneaten energy balls in the fridge and eat within a week.

TO FREEZE Freeze the energy balls on a baking tray so they don't stick together, then transfer to a rigid container. Defrost in the fridge.

Per ball: *113 cals*
2g protein   *9g carbs*
7g fat   *2g fibre*

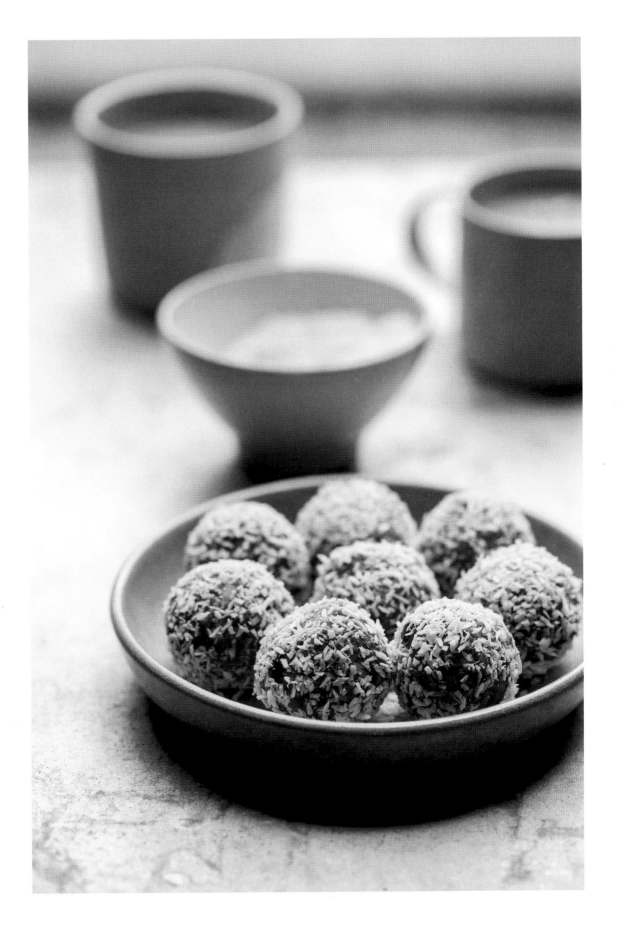

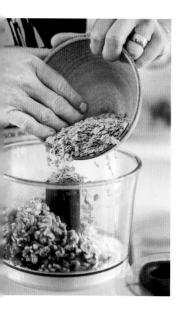
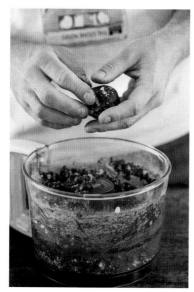
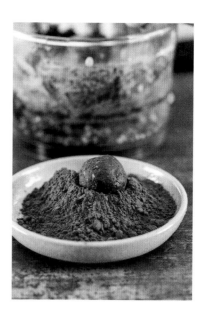
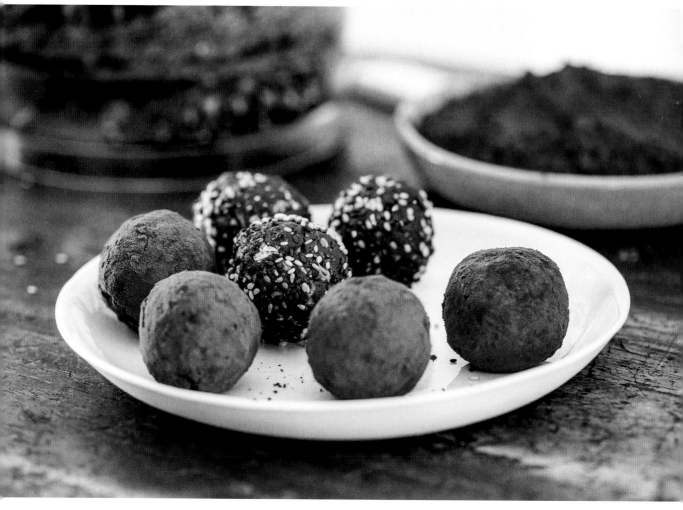

CHOCOLATE AND CRANBERRY ENERGY BALLS

I love the taste of sesame, and the intense flavour of tahini is the perfect addition to these little energy balls, which have a fantastic nutty quality. Rolling them in cocoa gives them a luxurious appearance – like posh chocolate truffles – and adds a lovely bitter-sweet edge. ♡ ❄

MAKES 20

200g Medjool dates, pitted
100ml boiling water
100g dried cranberries
80g good-quality cocoa powder, plus an extra 20g to finish
100g rolled oats
150g walnuts, toasted
60ml tahini
1 tbsp vanilla extract
1 tbsp honey

1 Cut the dates in half and place in a small heatproof bowl. Pour on the boiling water, cover and leave to soak for 10 minutes.

2 Put the rest of the ingredients into a food processor. Drain the dates in a sieve over a bowl to save the water. Add the dates to the food processor and pulse until well combined. If the mixture is too dry, add a little of the date water and pulse again.

3 Divide the mixture into 20 balls, each a bit larger than a golf ball. Roll each ball well, then roll in cocoa powder to coat lightly. Dust off any excess cocoa.

4 Place on a tray and refrigerate for 1 hour before serving. Store any uneaten energy balls in the fridge and eat within 10 days.

VARIATION For a crunchy-textured finish, roll the energy balls in 30g roasted mixed white and black sesame seeds instead of cocoa powder.

TO FREEZE Freeze the energy balls on a baking tray so they don't stick together, then transfer to a container. Defrost in the fridge.

Per ball: *157 cals*
4g protein   *15g carbs*
9g fat   *3g fibre*

SWEET

APRICOT FLAPJACK ENERGY BALLS

These tasty, oaty snacks are perfect to stash in your bag for a quick energy boost, either before or after a workout. ♡

MAKES 20

200g dried apricots, roughly chopped
100ml boiling water
50g dried apples
50g raisins
100g rolled oats
50g desiccated coconut
150g almonds, toasted
1 tsp ground cinnamon
1 tsp almond extract
1 tbsp vanilla extract
Grated zest of 1 lemon
2 tbsp honey

1 Place the dried apricots in a heatproof bowl and pour on the boiling water. Cover and leave to soak for 10 minutes.

2 Put the rest of the ingredients into a food processor. Drain the apricots in a sieve over a bowl to save the water. Add the apricots to the food processor and pulse until well combined. If the mixture is too dry, add a little of the apricot water and pulse again.

3 Divide the mixture into 20 balls, each a little larger than a golf ball, and roll each ball well so they're evenly sized.

4 Place on a tray and refrigerate for 1 hour before serving. Store any uneaten energy balls in the fridge and eat within 10 days.

TO FREEZE Freeze the energy balls on a baking tray so they don't stick together, then transfer to a rigid container. Defrost in the fridge.

 BONUS Made with all-natural ingredients, these are a much more nutritious option than most bought energy bars. They provide good carbs and lots of fibre, vitamins and minerals from the nuts and dried fruit.

SWEET

Per ball: *124 cals*
3g protein *12g carbs*
6g fat *3g fibre*

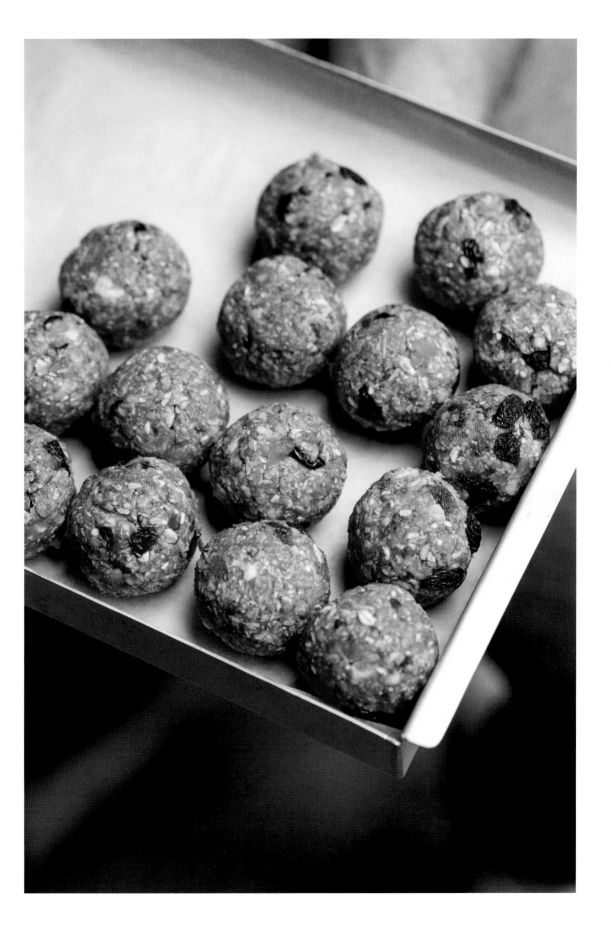

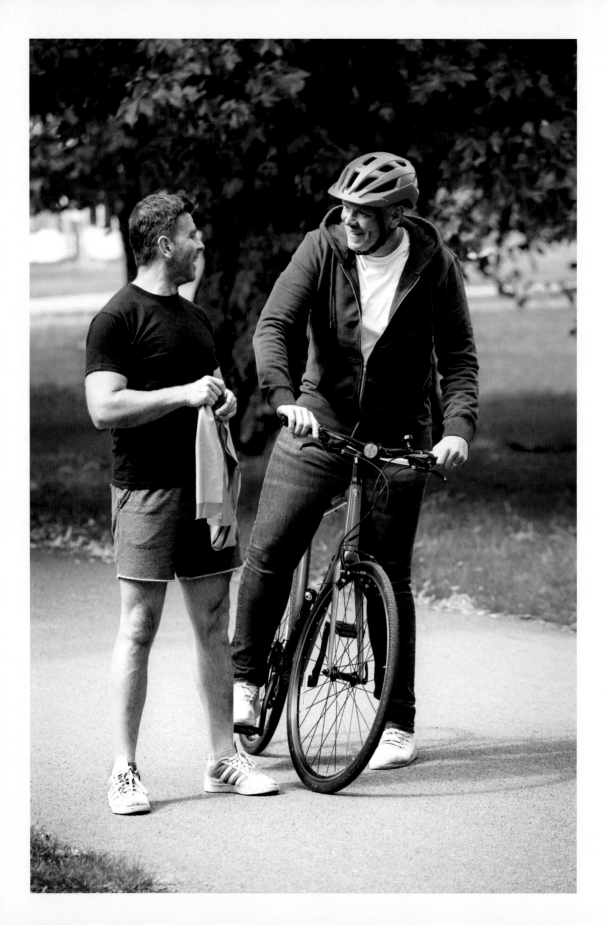

GET FIT WITH ADAM

Adam is a personal trainer who also has experience working as a rehabilitation instructor. I've known him since we were both studying in Cheltenham and he's still a really good mate of mine. Ads has done some truly amazing work helping people with serious medical conditions and rehabilitating individuals who have suffered life-changing injuries. He is the first person I call whenever I have a question about my fitness so I reckon he can help you on your own road to getting fit too – I'm going to hand you over to him now so he can talk you through the workout that he's put together especially for us…

Adam explains: The most important thing when it comes to exercise is that it needs to be regular and ideally enjoyable! Don't be scared of getting a little sweaty and always remember that whatever you manage to achieve is an amazing step in the right direction. Saying that, I know through my work as a personal trainer that people can always exercise more than they think they can – you really just need to be prepared to give it a go!

The NHS advises that adults aged between 19 and 64 should aim to complete 150 minutes of moderate cardio exercise each week, or 75 minutes of vigorous cardio exercise. Cardio (short for cardiovascular) exercise is basically anything that raises your heart rate, so moderate exercise includes things like brisk walking, riding a bike, basketball or going on a good hike, and vigorous exercise includes activities such as running and jogging, swimming quickly, football, rugby, tennis and skipping rope. Cardio is great for increasing heart health and burning calories; it can help improve your sleep and reduce stress, too – and it makes you feel good!

On top of your cardio workout, you need to include strength (also known as 'resistance') exercises on two or more days a week – such as lifting weights, working with resistance bands, or working with your own body weight, as you do in Pilates and yoga. Muscle strength is really important for overall good health and it helps build and maintain strong bones, which is especially important as we get older.

In addition, I highly recommend that you try to be more active whenever you can in your day-to-day life – most of us are guilty of sitting down a lot of the time, either at work or on the sofa in the evening. So look for ways to introduce more activity throughout your day – climbing the escalator rather than standing on it, or walking to town instead of hopping on a bus, for example. Even a short 10-minute stroll after eating can make a massive difference in controlling your blood-sugar levels.

On the following pages, I've put together a workout that has everything you need to stay fit and healthy. It's a really dynamic style of training, comprising bursts of cardiovascular activity coupled with resistance/strength-building exercises. I have seen amazing results with many of my personal training clients using this approach and have never once had any of them say that it's 'boring', so I hope you enjoy it too.

The workout may seem a little daunting to begin with, but I promise you that once you've performed it a handful of times it will become second nature. And if you can stick to this programme and fit it in 2 or 3 times a week (as well as keeping an eye on what you eat) you will see results. It will not only improve your fitness and strength, and help you shift a few pounds, but also make other activities you might enjoy, such as swimming or cycling, much easier – and you'll feel less knackered at work. Who doesn't want that?!

Unfortunately, we weren't able to hire a hunky model for the demo pics so you're left with me I'm afraid – I do apologise.

HOW IT WORKS

My workout is designed to be easy to follow and even easier to fit into your life. It has four components:

warm up • aerobic work • resistance work • cool down

All four of these are really important, so don't skip any of them.

The great thing about this workout is that the aerobic and resistance work are performed as a circuit so if you are really pushed for time or aren't able to manage the whole thing you can simply perform fewer circuits – you could even do some in the morning and some in the evening if you're super-dedicated. Remember to do the full warm up and cool down both times though!

If you are new to working out, or are a little deconditioned, then when it comes to the aerobic component of the workout, I recommend you begin by missing out every second move, with a 30-second rest in between each one, instead of doing all 8 moves. Then, as you build up your fitness, you can work towards completing all of the moves.

Start gradually, slowly but surely, working your way up to 4 full circuits in each session. I also advise speaking to a doctor before undertaking any new exercise programme, just to get the go-ahead. And if you're carrying a bit of extra timber, then I suggest that you go steady and be mindful of the more impact-based movements. Be as light as you can be on your feet – don't land flat-footed!

Finally, stick on whatever music makes you want to throw some shapes and then just get stuck in!

WHAT YOU'LL NEED

Working out at home is convenient, and you don't need a load of kit for it either. All you'll want is some comfortable clothing (including a good sports bra for women), a pair of well-fitting trainers to support your feet, a resistance band and something very sturdy to loop it around at floor height and also at head height – such as the end of your banisters or a leg of your bed. You'll also need a clock nearby or an interval app set up on your phone to keep you in check. One other tip is that you might get a better grip of the band or find it more comfortable if you wear a pair of PU palm work gloves or gardening gloves. These are by no means obligatory though!

Resistance bands are long and stretchy – a bit like giant elastic bands. When used as part of an exercise move, they add extra resistance, which requires your muscles to work harder. They usually come in packs of a few different strengths but can be doubled up if need be to increase their resistance. You can purchase them easily and cheaply online. Try to get bands that are hypoallergenic and at least 1.5–2 metres long. I think they are great because they offer a much more accessible alternative to using free weights – like dumbbells – and don't take up valuable space in your home. It's also really easy to adjust how much resistance they give, depending on where you are in your fitness journey. If you can't perform the exercises with a full range of movement then you might need to use a lighter band or alter the tension you are putting on it by holding the band in a different place.

THE WORKOUT

The workout overleaf counts towards your 75 minutes of vigorous cardio exercise each week and your resistance/strength exercises. Begin with the warm-up exercises to get your heart rate up and your muscles ready, then aim to complete the aerobic and resistance circuit four times, before finishing with the cool-down stretches.

You'll find explanations for how to do each move on pages 252–263. Everyone needs to ensure that they keep up good exercise technique so as to minimise the risk of injury. I can't stress this enough – technique is everything, so don't rush any of the moves and check your form regularly. It's always better to perform fewer beautiful reps than lots of ugly ones! Try to make it all the way through, but do obviously rest if and when you need to.

PUTTING IN EFFORT

The workout should take a maximum of 45 minutes to perform – any longer means you're not exercising at the right intensity. But don't charge through it like a bull in a china shop! Contrary to popular belief, you won't see results any more quickly and you increase the risk of injuring yourself.

The Rate of Perceived Exertion (RPE) scale

This will help you figure out the effort that you're putting in, depending on how easy you find it to talk while you're exercising. Each of the stages of the workout shows the RPE you should be aiming for. Be warned: you may appear a little bonkers if you're having a conversation with yourself the whole time you're working out. But who cares, just go for it!

1-2   **VERY EASY** You can talk with no effort

3   **EASY** You can talk with almost no effort

4   **MODERATELY EASY** You can talk comfortably with little effort

5   **MODERATE** Conversation requires some effort

6   **MODERATELY HARD** Conversation requires quite a bit of effort

7   **DIFFICULT** Conversation requires a lot of effort

8   **VERY DIFFICULT** Conversation requires maximum effort

9-10   **PEAK EFFORT** No-talking zone

WARM UP

See pages 252–3

	3½ minutes	RPE
Tiny steps	30 seconds	②❸
Low knee-raises	30 seconds	②❸
Marching	30 seconds	②❸
Side steps	30 seconds	②❸
Short side-lunges	30 seconds	②❸
Lunge with over-knee rotation	x 5	②❸
Squat to arm-swing	x 8	②❸

AEROBIC MOVES

See page 254

	4 minutes	RPE
Fast feet	30 seconds	⑤❻⑦
Marching (or rest)	30 seconds	②❸
Pogo jumps	30 seconds	⑤❻⑦
Side steps (or rest)	30 seconds	②❸
Shuffle jumps	30 seconds	⑤❻⑦
Marching (or rest)	30 seconds	②❸
Jumping jacks	30 seconds	⑤❻⑦
Side steps (or rest)	30 seconds	②❸

RESISTANCE MOVES

See pages 255–9

	5 minutes	**RPE**
Spear thruster	30 seconds each side	⑤ ⑥ ⑦
Face-pull and split-squat	30 seconds each side	⑤ ⑥ ⑦
Alternating side-lunge and chest-press	30 seconds each side	⑤ ⑥ ⑦
Reverse-lunge and row	30 seconds each side	⑤ ⑥ ⑦
Squat and shoulder-press	1 minute	⑤ ⑥ ⑦

Repeat the aerobic and resistance moves 3 more times

COOL DOWN

See pages 260–3

	4–6 minutes
Quads	15–20 seconds each side
Hamstrings	15–20 seconds each side
Hip flexors	15–20 seconds each side
Calves	15–20 seconds each side
Back	15–20 seconds each side
Chest	15–20 seconds each side
Biceps	15–20 seconds each side
Triceps	15–20 seconds each side

WARM UP

It's really important to warm up properly to get your muscles and joints ready for a workout. These are fun, easy warm-up moves where the main thing is just to get moving and get that heart rate up!

Tiny steps
Standing tall, walk on the spot with your feet barely leaving the ground.

Low knee-raises
Standing tall, walk on the spot, lifting your feet about 15–20cm off the ground. Introduce a small arm swing.

Marching (also known as high-knees)
Standing tall, march on the spot, lifting your feet 30–35cm off the ground. Swing your arms back and forth in time with your feet, with a 90° bend at the elbow.

Side steps
Standing tall, step one foot 60cm to the side, then bring it back to the middle to meet your other foot. Alternate each side.

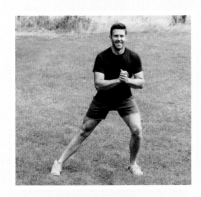

Short side-lunges
Stand tall. Step your left leg about 1 metre to the side, bending it at the knee. The toes of this foot should point at about 11 o'clock, so as to help prevent knee strain. The other leg should remain straight. The majority of your weight should be through the foot of the bent leg, but keep your weight back and try to ensure that your bent knee doesn't go over the end of your toes.

Pause, then return to your original position and repeat on the other side – the toes should point to 1 o'clock when you lunge with your right leg.

Continue to alternate between sides.

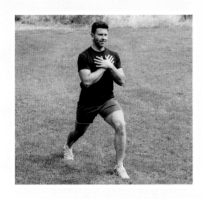 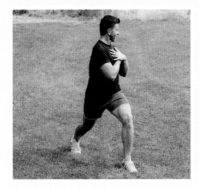

Lunge with over-knee rotation

Stand straight, then take a long step forwards with one leg. Your front leg should bend slightly at the knee with most of your weight equally distributed through the sole of the foot. Your back leg should be extended behind you with the heel off the floor. You will need to bend this knee slightly if you go deeper with your lunge.

Fold your arms across your chest, hands on shoulders. Now, rotate your body over your front leg.

Return to the centre then repeat four more times, before swapping sides.

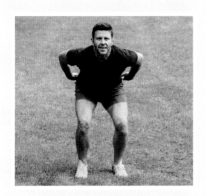 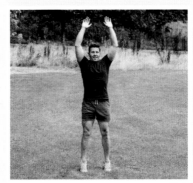

Squat to arm-swing

Come into a squat position, bending at the knees and hips and sticking your bottom and arms out behind you. Your feet must remain flat on the floor. Keep your hands close to your sides.

Now raise yourself up straight on to your toes and swing your arms up above your head – as if you're performing a Mexican wave!

Return to your squat position and repeat.

AEROBIC MOVES

Aerobic (cardio) exercise gets your heart rate up and your body moving! It's good for cardiovascular and respiratory health and is a fast-track to fitness. If you're a bit deconditioned or haven't exercised in a while, then start off by missing out every second exercise and take a 30-second rest instead; gradually build yourself up to the full sequence.

Fast feet
Standing tall, take tiny steps on the spot, as quickly as you can.

Marching
See page 252

Pogo jumps
Quick vertical jumps, taking off and landing on the balls of your feet and toes. Your feet barely leave the ground.

Side steps
See page 252

Shuffle jumps
Tiny step-jumps back and forth. Use a normal stride length that feels comfortable for you. And don't jump too high – your feet should just clear the floor.

Marching
See page 252

Jumping jacks
Good old-fashioned star jumps! Start by standing with your feet together and your arms down by your sides. Jump vertically and make a star shape with your arms and legs – you only need leave the ground by 6–8cm.

Side steps
See page 252

RESISTANCE MOVES

Strength exercises are important for building and maintaining good muscle development and bone health. Here we use resistance bands (see page 248), which require your muscles to work harder. Use a strength of band that gives you a good workout, but still allows you to complete the moves with a full range of movement. Attach your resistance band to something sturdy when required.

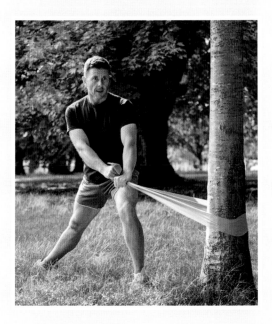 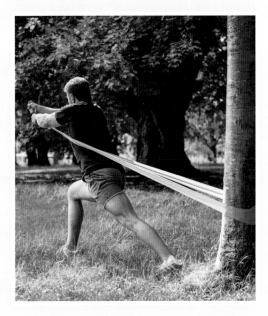

Spear thruster

This is a great dynamic exercise, which really focuses the mind and body. It works the back, chest, arms, quads, core, glutes and adductors.

Loop the resistance band around something sturdy and near to the ground and then step away, holding the band firmly so it becomes taut.

Adopt a side-lunge stance (see page 252) of about 1.5 metres while holding on to the end of the band with both hands. Your hands should be level with the hip nearest where the band is attached.

Pull the band across your body and then push it away, as if thrusting a spear. Your weight should shift from your back leg to your front one.

Return to the start position, then repeat.

Once your 30 seconds is up, repeat on the other side.

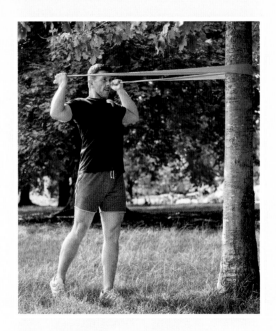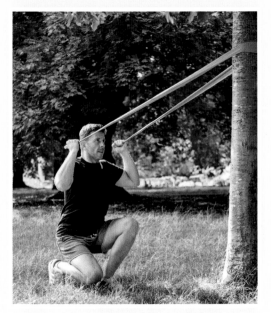

Face-pull and split-squat

The 'face-pull and split-squat' is a must for those of us who spend a lot of time slouched over computers, phones or tablets, as it can help improve your posture. This move works your mid and upper back, rotator cuff, glutes, quads and calves.

Loop the resistance band around something sturdy, like a bannister rail, at head height.

Take a 'split stance', which is similar to a long stride backwards; your back heel should be off the ground. Take hold of the band at each end, with your palms facing inwards and your elbows bent. Pull the band towards your face – your hands should travel either side of your head and finish further back than your elbow.

Slowly return your hands to their original position.

Come into a split squat position, sticking your bottom out and bending both knees. Keep the band at shoulder height. The main bulk of your weight should be through the heel of your front foot – try not to let that knee go too far over the toes.

Drive through the lead leg and come up to standing, then resume your original position before repeating.

Once your 30 seconds is up, repeat on the other side.

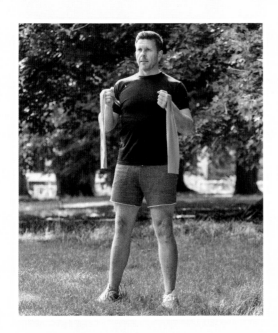
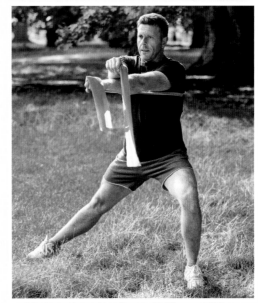

Alternating side-lunge and chest-press

We spend 99% of our lives travelling in the same forward direction – go crab for once! This move works your chest, triceps, front deltoids, abductors, adductors, glutes and hamstrings.

Start with your feet a little more than hip width apart. Loop the resistance band around your back, holding it with the palms facing inwards and your elbows bent, so that you can take an equal length in each hand.

Stand tall. Step your left leg about 1–1.5 metres to the side, bending it at the knee. The toes of this leg should point at about 11 o'clock, so as to help prevent knee strain. The other leg should remain straight. The majority of your weight should be through the foot of the bent leg, but keep your weight back and try to ensure that your bent knee doesn't go over the end of your toes.

Press your arms forward and while keeping them straight, cross your right arm over the left arm so that your elbows align.

Bring your arms back and return to the starting position. Repeat, alternating legs and arms. The toes should point to 1 o'clock when you lunge with your right leg.

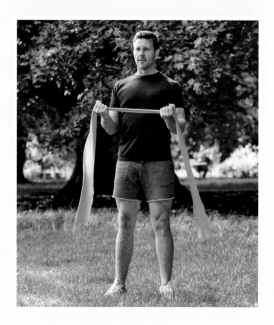 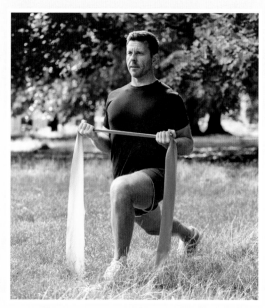

Reverse-lunge and row

This is a superb way to build overall body strength while improving your balance and coordination. It works your mid back, rotator cuff, biceps, quads, glutes and calves.

Stand straight, with your elbows bent at a 90° angle. Keep your elbows tight to the side of your body.

Grip the resistance band in front of you with your palms facing upwards and about 20cm apart.

Lunge backwards with one leg but keep the heel off the floor – bend your front leg at the same time. The main bulk of your weight should be through the front leg – you may need to bend forward slightly at your hips.

Pull the band apart 5–8cm but keep your elbows close to the sides of your body.

Draw the band back towards the top of your tummy and squeeze the muscles in your back.

Bring the band forward again while maintaining the tension in it. Return to your start position then repeat the move.

Once your 30 seconds is up, swap legs.

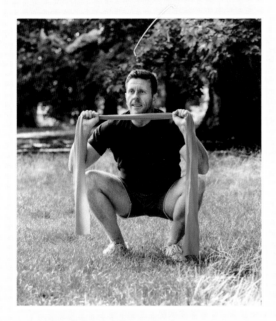 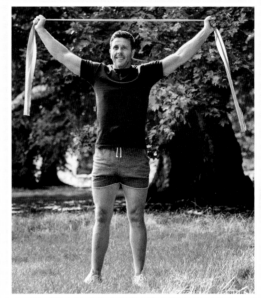

Squat and shoulder-press

Here is a classic move that will never get old. It works your shoulders, core, triceps, glutes, quads and hamstrings.

Stand straight with your feet shoulder-width apart. Your toes should point a few centimetres outward, not straight ahead.

With your palms facing forward, hold a section of the resistance band up near your chest, slightly more than shoulder width apart.

Bend at the knees and hips, sticking your bottom out, as you come down slowly into a squat. Keep your heels on the ground.

Stand up and stretch your arms above your head while pulling the resistance band apart.

Bring the band back down to your chest and return to your start position. Repeat.

COOL DOWN

It's important that you cool down and perform some static stretches at the end of each workout. This will help ease any muscle aches and stiffness. A little achiness is to be expected, especially if you're not used to exercising. However, if you feel sharp nagging joint pain or your muscles are actually painful, then this is a sign that you're either doing too much, your form is off, or that the exercises aren't suitable for you.

Your muscles can actually feel more achy a couple of days after you've trained rather than on the day immediately following your workout, so be prepared. To help prevent this, always do a proper warm up and cool down, and if your muscles do feel sore then undertake some extra, less strenuous activity such as walking or swimming to loosen them up.

Work your way through these static stretches for at least 2 minutes, being careful not to overstretch or bounce while you're doing them.

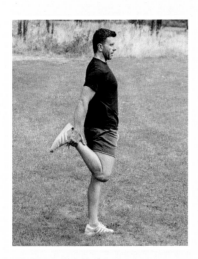

Quads

Stand on your left leg (you can hold on to a chair or a wall for balance with your right hand if you need to).

From behind you, grab your right foot with your right hand, bringing your heel in towards your bottom. Push your hips forwards.

Hold for 15–20 seconds, then repeat on the other side.

Hamstrings

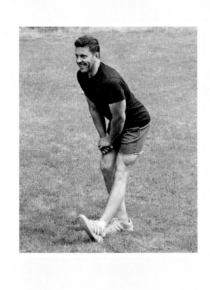

Stretch one leg out in front of you while slightly bending the supporting leg. The outstretched foot needs to have its toes up and its heel on the floor.

Place your hands just above the knee of the bent leg to support yourself. Lean forwards from your hips while maintaining a straight back. You should feel a stretch down the back of the straight leg.

Hold for 15–20 seconds, then repeat on the other side.

Hip flexors

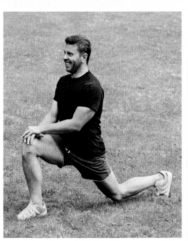

Take a really nice long lunge forward and place your hands just above the bent knee.

While keeping your torso upright – gently lower yourself down so that you feel a stretch across the groin area of the back leg.

Hold for 15–20 seconds, then repeat on the other side.

Calves

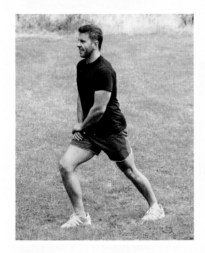

Adopt a short lunge position, with your front right leg bent and your back left leg straight. Keep both feet flat on the ground, toes pointing forwards. Your weight should be through the front leg.

Place your hands on the top of your front leg to help you balance. You should feel a stretch through the calf of your back leg.

Hold for 15–20 seconds, then repeat on the other side.

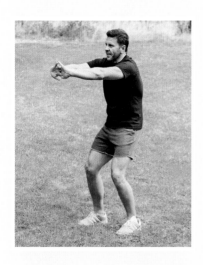

Back

Bending your knees, lock your fingers together and then push your hand out in front of you, palms first.

Slouch your shoulders so that you feel the stretch across your back.

Hold for 15–20 seconds.

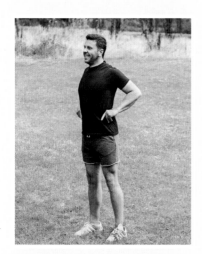

Chest

Place your hands on your hips.

Gently push back your elbows and push your chest forward.

Hold for 15–20 seconds.

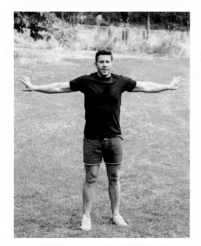

Biceps

Stand nice and tall with your arms stretched out to either side at shoulder height.

With your palms facing out, push your thumbs down and back.

Hold for 15–20 seconds.

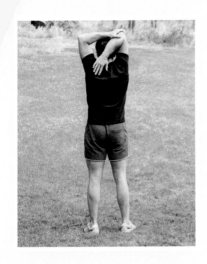

Triceps

Standing straight, reach your right arm over and behind your head, aiming to touch the opposite shoulder blade.

Place your left hand on the bent right elbow and then gently push the elbow against it – you should feel the stretch down the back of the arm.

Hold for 15–20 seconds, then repeat on the other side.

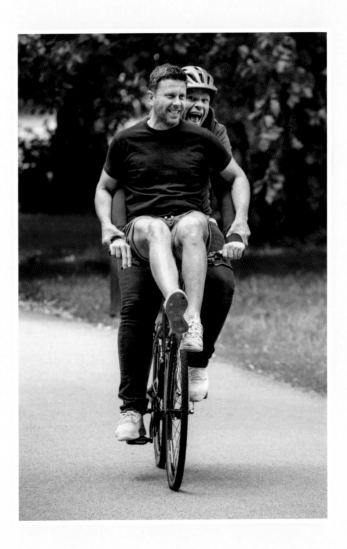

INDEX

meat 190–1
  see also beef, lamb *etc*
meatballs, turkey 180–1
melon and mint sorbet 231
milk: berry and yoghurt
  breakfast shake 59
  mocha 'get up and go' shake
  60
  nutty banana breakfast
  shake 56
mint: melon and mint sorbet
  231
  minted peas 142
minute steaks with kale 211
miso: chicken, miso and
  mushroom ramen 174–5
  miso stir-fried greens with
  fried egg 110
mixed berry crumble 228
mocha 'get up and go' shake
  60
monkfish and coconut curry
  152
muffins, breakfast 54
mushrooms: baked ricotta-
  stuffed mushrooms 108
  beef ragu with pasta 208–9
  chicken, miso and mushroom
  ramen 174–5
  cottage pie 202–4
  roasted mushroom-stuffed
  peppers 119
mustard pork 198

N
noodles: chicken, miso and
  mushroom ramen 174–5
  chicken noodle soup 170
  chicken pho 173
nuoc cham 79
nuts *see* hazelnuts, walnuts *etc*
nutty banana breakfast shake
  56

O
oats: apple and cardamom
  overnight oats 26
  apricot flapjack energy balls
  242
  banana and pecan nut
  porridge 30
  berry and yoghurt breakfast
  shake 59

breakfast muffins 54
carrot cake energy balls 238
chocolate and cranberry
  energy balls 241
mixed berry crumble 228
mocha 'get up and go' shake
  60
nutty banana breakfast shake
  56
peach Melba overnight oats
  24
okra: prawn and okra curry
  155
omelettes: chicken and leek
  baked omelette 38
  salmon and avocado
  egg-white omelette 42
onions: beef ragu with pasta
  208–9
  cottage pie 202–4
  pickled red onion 92
  roast onion, chickpea and
  halloumi salad 122
  smoky beef chilli 197
oranges: fruit compote 225
oven-baked fish fingers 142–3

P
pancakes: Chinese-style
  chicken pancakes 169
  tahini and honey pancakes
  53
pancetta: smoked pancetta
  and lentil soup 102
panna cottas, Earl Grey 225
paprika chicken 184
parsnips: root vegetable
  boulangère 120
passion fruit: strawberry and
  passion fruit chia pots 35
pasta: beef ragu with pasta
  208–9
  cavolo nero penne 114
  spinach and ricotta pasta
  bake 126–7
pastries: chicken and spinach
  baked samosas 76
pastry 156–7
pâté, smoked mackerel 68
peach Melba overnight oats 24
peanut butter: peanut dipping
  sauce 79
pearl barley *see* barley

pears: fruit compote 225
  pear and ginger loaf cake
  234
peas: cottage pie 202–4
  lamb and barley stew 206
  minted peas 142
  pea pesto 144
  pork loin with celeriac, garlic
  and cider 214
pecan nuts: banana and pecan
  nut porridge 30
  carrot cake energy balls 238
  crunchy nut butter 48
peppers: beans in tomato
  sauce 186–8
  beef ragu with pasta 208–9
  black bean and butternut
  chilli 113
  black pepper beef stir-fry
  192
  chicken ratatouille 179
  corn and black bean burrito
  bowls 92
  dirty rice 96, 99
  lamb bhuna 200
  roast onion, chickpea and
  halloumi salad 122
  roasted mushroom-stuffed
  peppers 119
  roasted pepper sauce 180–1
  smoky beef chilli 197
  Spanish-style eggs with
  chorizo 41
  spicy Mexican-style bean
  burger 116
  spinach and ricotta pasta
  bake 126–7
peri peri chicken 96
pesto, pea 144
pho, chicken 173
pickles: pickled radishes 90
  pickled red onion 92
  quick cucumber pickle 68
pilaf: chicken, brown rice and
  lentil 182
pineapple: 'get your greens in'
  smoothie 63
pinto beans: Spanish-style
  eggs with chorizo 41
planning 19
plum sauce 169
pogo jumps, aerobic exercise
  254

smoked pancetta and lentil
soup 102
Spanish-style eggs with
chorizo 41
spear thruster, resistance
exercise 255
spinach: chicken and spinach
baked samosas 76
chicken and yoghurt curry
176
'get your greens in' smoothie
63
green eggs and ham 44
quick black dhal 128
spinach and ricotta pasta
bake 126–7
spinach salad 71
squash *see* butternut squash
squat and shoulder-press,
resistance exercise 259
squat to arm-swing exercise
253
squid, chickpea and chorizo
stew 150
steak tacos with burnt corn
salsa 194
stews: beef ragu with pasta
208–9
lamb and barley stew 206
squid, chickpea and chorizo
stew 150
stir-fries: black pepper beef
stir-fry 192
Sichuan beef and broccoli
stir-fry 212
tofu stir-fry 125
strawberries: rhubarb compote
29
strawberry and passion fruit
chia pots 35
strength exercises 12, 245
swede: root vegetable
boulangère 120
sweet potatoes: carrot and
quinoa fritters 71
chicken tagine traybake 163
cottage pie 202–4
oven-baked fish fingers
142–3
roast pumpkin and sweet
potato soup 131
root vegetable boulangère
120

sweetcorn: corn and black
bean burrito bowls 92
tofu stir-fry 125
tuna cobb salad bowl 95
see also corn-on-the-cob
swimming 12

T

tacos: spiced fish tacos 134
steak tacos with burnt corn
salsa 194
tahini: tahini and honey
pancakes 53
tahini yoghurt 53
tartare sauce 142–3
tea: Earl Grey panna cottas
225
Lady Grey quinoa porridge
with blueberries 32
teriyaki salmon 90
Thai fish cakes 141
tiny steps, warm-up exercise
252
toast, chilli avocado 47
tofu stir-fry 125
tomatoes: beans in tomato
sauce 186–8
beef ragu with pasta 208–9
black bean and butternut
chilli 113
burnt corn salsa 194
chicken ratatouille 179
chicken, tomato and
mozzarella salad 160
chilli avocado toast 47
cottage pie 202–4
lamb bhuna 200
smoked pancetta and lentil
soup 102
smoky beef chilli 197
Spanish-style eggs with
chorizo 41
spinach and ricotta pasta
bake 126–7
squid, chickpea and chorizo
stew 150
tomato salsa 134
tortillas: spiced fish tacos 134
steak tacos with burnt corn
salsa 194
triceps, cooling-down exercise
263
tuna cobb salad bowl 95

turkey 158–9
quinoa turkey schnitzels 166
turkey meatballs in roasted
pepper sauce 180–1
turkey sausages and beans
186–8
turnips: lamb and barley stew
206

V

vegetables: crudités 68
see also peppers, tomatoes
etc

W

walnuts: carrot cake energy
balls 238
chocolate and cranberry
energy balls 241
crunchy nut butter 48
mixed berry crumble 228
warm-up exercises 250, 252–3
water, drinking 11
wholemeal soda bread rolls
105
workout, exercise 245–63

Y

yoghurt: apple and cardamom
overnight oats 26
berry and yoghurt breakfast
shake 59
blackberry and yoghurt fool
220
chicken and yoghurt curry
176
chocolate and raspberry
cupcakes 237
Earl Grey panna cottas 225
harissa yoghurt 164
lemon and blueberry yoghurt
pots 222
peach Melba overnight oats
24
strawberry and passion fruit
chia pots 35
tahini yoghurt 53

THANKS!

Firstly I would like to say a huge thank you to all of Bloomsbury Publishing and Absolute Press. Nigel Newton, Natalie Bellos, Xa Shaw Stewart, Jon Croft, Nicola Hill, Amanda Shipp, Ellen Williams, Donough Shanahan, Trâm-Anh Doan, Laura Brodie: you guys are the dream publishing team, warm, understanding, creative and kind. Working alongside the Bloomsbury crew, I want to give massive high fives to these guys for editing, nutritional guidance, design, illustration and recipe testing: Janet Illsley, Anita Bean, David Eldridge and Yoko Yamaguchi at Two Associates, Frankie Unsworth, Sophie Mackinnon and Christina Mackenzie. Thank you.

Fist bumps all round for food and photos. Starting with the forever fantastic Cristian Barnett for continuing to make this food look at home and accessible, but at the same time beautiful. To my amazing Australian mate, Nicole Herft: you constantly bring energy, enthusiasm and incredible cooking for us to work with. Your top drawer team of food stylists, Holly Cochrane, Rosie Mackean and Alex Gray, really made this book shoot. To Chris Mackett, thanks for being my stunt double, covering my back and making sure that everything we do is built on the foundation we made 17 years ago, back when we started this journey together. Love you mate. Big thank you to Lydia McPherson and Lauren Law for all the beautiful ceramics, props and styling.

To the *Lose Weight & Get Fit* TV gang, I want to say a massive thank you to the volunteers who put themselves in front of the camera and opened themselves up to the scrutiny of the British public, inspiring everybody. Alex Redworth, Dan Bunce, Bev Smith, Mumtaz Kadodia, Chris Jenkinson, Luke Roberts, Lauren Baker, Emma Adams, Manny Masih, Maxine Smith and Sandie Mills: you guys really are amazing to work with, and also make me very proud.

To everybody at Bone Soup, thank you for all your hard work and making the show look so great. Rich Bowron, Sarah Myland, Joanna Boyle, Richard Hill, Sophie Wells, Rosa Brough, Louise Maynard, Jack Coathupe, Chris Hayes, Niall Newport, Robbie Johnson, Nick Murray, Miranda Pincott, Jessica Parrish, Lucy Kattenhorn, Christopher White, Chris Mallett, Cath Hunter, Bobby Tutton, Georgia May, Gemma Stoddart and Jon Hubbard: you guys are the best. It was incredibly well thought out behind the scenes – from research at the top level through to direction and vision, every detail was picked through and, more importantly, every person was cared for. The show also sounds good (thanks, Robbie Johnson). I'd also like to give a massive thank you to David Brindley and Michael Jochnowitz at the BBC for commissioning the series.

A big shout out to the guys who make my life run. First and foremost (and the first time her name will be in a book with this particular surname), Alex Reilly. I don't know what I'd do without you, and I don't think anyone else would know what to do with me if you weren't there! Borra Garson, Louise Leftwich, Gemma Bell and the rest of the agent's and PR teams, thanks for getting me stuff, and making sure I don't say silly things!

Now the hugs go out to my home life. The people who on a daily basis keep allowing me to be me. To the personal trainers who make me work hard if I have a cake, Dino Bonwick and Adam Peacock. Thanks chaps for making me sweat and spend hours every week hating the sound of your voice, but loving the results, ha ha ha! To Suze, for helping to relieve parental guilt; I am sorry I taught him that burping is funny... and that I can't stop it happening now! To Katie, thanks for keeping domestic dramas to a minimum. And to Sammy and Ryan for making sure that the dogs don't wee inside!

To the ever-growing, incredibly inspiring and brilliantly loyal pub and restaurant teams. You guys deserve so many plaudits, medals of honour and rosettes, I don't know where to begin. The dedication that you show to consistency leads to growth in all areas of the business and I can't thank you enough. Every single one of you is so special. Thank you all at The Hand and Flowers, The Coach, Kerridge's Bar & Grill, The Butcher's Tap, The Bull & Bear and Lush by Tom Kerridge. There are too many of you to individually thank at the back of this book, but fist bumps to you all. You are only as good as the team you surround yourself with, and I really am surrounded by the best people.

And finally, Bef and Ace-man. Thank you for being so understanding, even if one of you doesn't really understand because you're 4 years old.

BLOOMSBURY ABSOLUTE

Bloomsbury Publishing Plc

50 Bedford Square, London, WC1B 3DP, UK

BLOOMSBURY, BLOOMSBURY ABSOLUTE,
the Diana logo and the Absolute Press logo are
trademarks of Bloomsbury Publishing Plc

First published in Great Britain 2019

Text © Tom Kerridge, 2019

Photography © Cristian Barnett, 2019

Illustrations © David Eldridge,
    Two Associates, 2019

Tom Kerridge, Cristian Barnett and David Eldridge,
Two Associates, have asserted their right under the
Copyright, Designs and Patents Act, 1988, to be
identified as author, photographer and illustrator,
respectively, of this work.

BBC and the BBC logo are trademarks of the
British Broadcasting Corporation and are used
under licence. BBC logo © BBC 1996.

For legal purposes, the acknowledgements
on pages 270–1 constitute an extension of this
copyright page.

All rights reserved. No part of this publication may
be reproduced or transmitted in any form or by
any means, electronic or mechanical, including
photocopying, recording, or any information
storage or retrieval system, without prior
permission in writing from the publishers.

The information contained in this book is provided
by way of general guidance in relation to the
specific subject matters addressed herein, but it
is not a substitute for specialist dietary advice.
It should not be relied on for medical, health-care,
pharmaceutical or other professional advice on
specific dietary or health needs. This book is sold
with the understanding that the author and
publisher are not engaged in rendering medical,
health or any other kind of personal or professional
services. The reader should consult a competent
medical or health professional before adopting any
of the suggestions in this book or drawing
inferences from it.

The author and publisher specifically disclaim, as
far as the law allows, any responsibility from any
liability, loss or risk (personal or otherwise) which
is incurred as a consequence, directly or indirectly,
of the use and applications of any of the contents
of this book. If you are on medication of any
description, please consult your doctor or health
professional before embarking on any fast or diet.

A catalogue record for this book is available from
the British Library

ISBN: HB: 978-1-4729-6282-9
       eBook: 978-1-4729-6283-6

10 9 8 7 6 5 4 3 2 1

Project Editor: Janet Illsley
Nutritional Consultant: Anita Bean
Design: Two Associates
Photographs: Cristian Barnett
Food Styling: Nicole Herft
Art Direction and Styling: Lydia McPherson
Illustrations: Two Associates
Indexer: Hilary Bird

Thanks to the following for their ceramics:
Homefolk Ceramics
www.homefolkceramics.com

Rosie Livemore
www.herclay.com
@_herclay_

Sinikka Harms Ceramics
www.sinikkaharms.de
@sinikkaharmsceramics

Printed and bound in Germany by Mohn Media

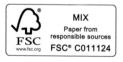

FSC
www.fsc.org

MIX
Paper from
responsible sources
FSC® C011124

To find out more about our authors and books
visit www.bloomsbury.com and sign up for our
newsletters

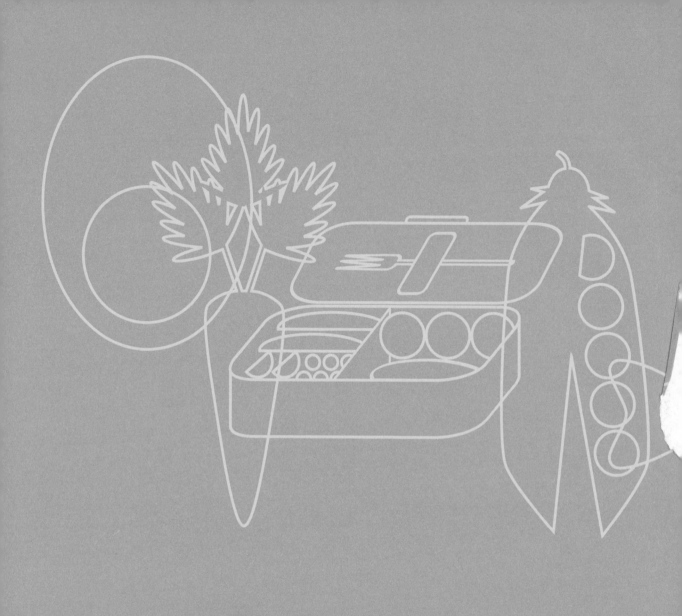